LIVING THERAPY SERIES

Workplace Counselling in the NHS

Person-Centred Dialogues

Richard Bryant-Jefferies

Radcliffe Publishing
Oxford • Seattle

Radcliffe Publishing Ltd
18 Marcham Road
Abingdon
Oxon OX14 1AA
United Kingdom

www.radcliffe-oxford.com
Electronic catalogue and worldwide online ordering facility.

British Library Cataloguing in Publication Data

A catalogue record for this book is available from the British Library.

ISBN 1 85775 727 0

Typeset by Aarontype Ltd, Easton, Bristol
Printed and bound by TJ International Ltd, Padstow, Cornwall

Contents

Foreword

Working in a stressful environment is bad for your health and increases accidents. In recent years this has been recognised and steps have been taken to reduce the physical and psychosocial hazards that cause stress at work. However, there will always be some stress at work and it is therefore important to understand how much is an essential part of day-to-day activities associated with getting the job done and how much is unnecessary or imported from outside the workplace.

The benefits of workplace counselling have recently been illustrated in a major study by Professor John McLeod in *A Systematic Study of the Research Evidence: the facts* where he reviewed over 80 studies covering the experiences of 10 000 clients over 45 years. Thus, it is clear that many companies and organisations now recognise the need for stress counselling. For example, Astra Zeneca offers its workforce a confidential programme of Counselling and Life Management (CaLM) (Corporate Responsibility Report 2003).

A recent study on managing the risk of work-related stress by Clarke and Cooper (2004) suggests three levels of management intervention to reduce stress. Primary, where the action is preventative and aimed at the work environment; secondary, where the interventions have a preventative/reactive nature aimed at improving responses to stressors through, for example, stress management training; and tertiary, where the focus is on the treatment of employees already suffering illness. All these are aimed at minimising the damage done by stress and use employee assistance programmes or offer in-house stress counselling.

Stress counselling in the workplace is at the heart of Richard Bryant-Jefferies' latest book, and he has chosen to locate his timely and informative study in the NHS.

The NHS is the largest single employer in Europe and it is undergoing radical change due to the introduction of many new policies and targets, as well as the new pay scales and terms and conditions of service for staff covered in 'Agenda for Change', which became operational on 1 December 2004. All this is having a stressful impact on much of its workforce. Change, with its associated stress, is not new to NHS employees. Over its history political decisions have been taken that have resulted in numerous documents outlining ways to improve the NHS and, ultimately, services to patients. All of which is commendable but the implementation of such initiatives, usually within a short timeframe, has not been without cost to NHS managers and other healthcare staff.

Richard Bryant-Jefferies shows an understanding of these stresses and strains, demonstrated through his case presentation. His style of writing is successful because it speaks of the real experience of counsellors. Although the workplace setting may be unfamiliar to the reader, it is likely that they will recognise the situations and will have had clients who have experienced some of the problems he illustrates. He manages to bring his cases alive in such a way as to enable the reader to be an invisible observer of the counselling process. This allows the practitioner to compare and contrast his or her own practice with the work of the counsellor in the case studies. For example, an exchange between one of the counsellors and his supervisor using the person-centred approach was useful to me and illuminating for my own practice.

I enjoyed reading this book and hope that you get as much out of it as I did. The author has a clear, informative and accessible style and his way of presenting material will be of special interest to trainers and trainees because it is rooted in a particular theory and practice, and arises out of his clinical experience. It builds on his previous work and leads one to hope for further explorations in this field.

Pat Seber
April 2005

Pat Seber has had a varied counselling career. Her first introduction to counselling was with Relate. She then moved on to managing services within the voluntary and private sector. Pat has a long association with the NHS as an employee and a private practitioner in both primary and secondary care. She is currently employed by a Mental Health Trust as lead counsellor and manager for a Primary Care Counselling Service in central Liverpool. Previously she worked in a large teaching hospital where she set up and ran a counselling service for pregnant women. Pat is a Fellow of the British Association for Counselling and Psychotherapy (BACP) and Deputy Chair of the Faculty of Healthcare Counsellors and Psychotherapists (FHCP), the Healthcare Division of BACP. Within FHCP she has the role of Employment Advisor and has worked closely with Unison in the preparation and development of profiles for counsellors employed in the NHS as part of 'Agenda for Change'. She holds a Masters degree in Counselling.

References

Astra Zeneca (2003) *Counselling and Life Management: CaLM* (Corporate Responsibility Report). Astra Zeneca.

Clarke S and Cooper CL (2004) *Managing the Risk of Workplace Stress: Health and Safety Hazards.* Routledge, London.

McLeod J (2001, modified 2004) *Counselling in the Workplace. A Systematic Study of the Research Evidence: the facts.* BACP, Rugby and School of Social and Health Sciences, University of Abertay, Dundee.

Preface

The aim of the *Living Therapy* series is to offer the reader an opportunity to experience and to appreciate, through the use of dialogue, some of the diverse and challenging issues that can arise during counselling (Bryant-Jefferies, 2003a, b; 2004). The success of the preceding books, and the appreciative comments received from readers and independent reviewers, is encouragement enough to seek to extend this style into other issues and areas of person-centred counselling. Again and again people remark on how readable these books are, how much they bring the therapeutic process alive. In particular, students of counselling and psychotherapy have remarked on how accessible the text is. Trainers and others who are experienced in the field have indicated to me the timeliness of a series that focuses the application of the person-centred approach to working therapeutically with clients having particular issues. This is both heartening and encouraging. I want the style to draw people into the narrative and feel engaged with the characters and the therapeutic process. I want this series to be what I would term 'an experiential read'.

As with the other books in the *Living Therapy* series (Radcliffe Publishing), this book is composed of fictitious dialogues between fictitious clients and their counsellors, both working in the NHS, and between the counsellors and their supervisors. Within the dialogues are woven the reflective thoughts and feelings of the clients, the counsellors and the supervisors, along with boxed comments on the process and references to person-centred theory. I do not seek to provide all the answers. Rather I want to convey something of the process of working with representative material that can arise so that the reader may be stimulated into processing their own reactions, and reflecting on the relevance and effectiveness of the therapeutic responses, to thereby gain insight into themselves and their practice. Often it will simply lead to more questions which I hope will prove stimulating to the reader and encourage them to think through their own theoretical, philosophical and ethical positions and their boundary of competence.

Recent years have seen a tremendous growth in the number of organisations that have developed counselling facilities for staff. Some have employed their own counsellor or counsellors, to work with staff members, others have contracted out to agencies offering 'Employee Assistance Programmes'. These services are a response to the recognition that staff are affected by experiences related to their work (and sometimes linked to difficulties from outside of work) and that the most constructive way forward is to offer therapeutic assistance to help them resolve the problems and once again contribute to the organisation.

The NHS has been chosen as the setting for the counsellor and client in this title in the *Living Therapy* series for a number of reasons. First, the NHS is the largest UK employer. It is an organisation in which staff may feel they have very little say in what goes on as directives come from so far above, and it seems to be in a constant state of flux. Compared with other workplace settings, employees are under an extra level of strain that comes from dealing with patients and families at very stressful times in their lives. It also employs a tremendous range of professionals who are required to work together within the NHS healthcare system, and has an ethnic mix probably greater than any other employing organisation in the UK. It brings together people from so many personal and professional backgrounds and for the counsellor there has to be a readiness and an ability to work with clients from all levels of the organisation, on a range of issues that affect their NHS workplace performance.

In their report for The Nuffield Provincial Hospitals Trust, Williams *et al.* (1998) highlighted the significantly high levels of psychological distress experienced by the doctors, nurses and managers, and the risks that this, in turn, posed not only for the staff themselves, but also the service and the patients. The Report draws attention to areas of particular concern, which have been summarised in the Department of Health's guidance entitled *The Provision of Counselling Services for Staff in the NHS* as follows.

- Stress in health service staff is substantially higher than in employees in general in the United Kingdom.
- NHS managers are twice as likely to be above the threshold for psychological distress as other British managers.
- New stressors are occurring with the perceived rise of violence to staff and with fears of contamination by HIV/HEP. B/C.
- Nursing and medicine have some of the highest rates of suicide amongst professional staff groups.
- Stress at work is a widespread problem not only for nurses and doctors but also for managers (DoH, 2000, p. 7).

The Nuffield Report (Williams *et al.*, 1998) also highlighted the high human and financial costs, and the positive fact that many NHS trusts were establishing counselling services as a result of concerns for staff health, welfare and the high and increasing levels of stress. The provision of counselling services has become more widespread within the NHS in line with meeting the target in the NHS Human Resources Framework, *Working Together: securing a quality workforce for the NHS*, for all NHS staff to have access to counselling services by April 2000. Increasing numbers of staff can now gain access to an NHS workplace scheme. The actual nature of the counselling services that have been established varies from site to site. Some, as mentioned above, buy in outside agencies, some set-up their own services and employ new staff, still others use existing staff with the necessary skills, to run the counselling service.

Workplace Counselling in the NHS: person-centred dialogues is intended as much for experienced workplace counsellors as it is for trainees. It provides real insight into what can occur during counselling sessions. I hope it will raise awareness of, and inform, not only person-centred practice within this context, but also contribute to other theoretical approaches within the world of counselling, psychotherapy, and the various branches of psychology. Reflections on the therapeutic process and points for discussion are included to stimulate further thought and debate. Included in this book is material to inform the training process of counsellors and others who seek to work in the NHS setting.

Workplace Counselling in the NHS: person-centred dialogues is an essential resource for NHS managers, supervisors, team leaders and human resources staff, providing them with greater insight and understanding of the counselling process, from a person-centred theoretical perspective. It will have value, too, for the many professionals from all healthcare and allied services working within the NHS who may themselves be feeling a need to seek workplace counselling. The text demystifies what can occur in therapy within an NHS context. The issues presented are relevant to the NHS as it stands today, and affect everyone who works within it, at whatever level and in whatever speciality.

Richard Bryant-Jefferies
April 2005

About the author

Richard Bryant-Jefferies qualified as a person-centred counsellor/therapist in 1994 and remains passionate about the application and effectiveness of this approach. Between early 1995 and mid-2003 Richard worked at a community drug and alcohol service in Surrey as an alcohol counsellor. Since 2003 he has worked for the Central and North West London Mental Health NHS Trust, managing substance misuse service within the Royal Borough of Kensington and Chelsea in London. He has experience of offering both counselling and supervision in NHS, GP and private settings, and has provided training through 'alcohol awareness and response' workshops. He also offers workshops based on the use of written dialogue as a contribution to continuing professional development and within training programmes. His website address is: www.bryant-jefferies. freeserve.co.uk

Richard had his first book on a counselling theme published in 2001, *Counselling the Person Beyond the Alcohol Problem* (Jessica Kingsley Publishers), providing theoretical yet practical insights into the application of the person-centred approach within the context of the 'cycle of change' model that has been widely adopted to describe the process of change in the field of addiction. Since then he was been writing for the *Living Therapy* series, producing an on-going series of person-centred dialogues: *Problem Drinking, Time Limited Therapy in Primary Care, Counselling a Survivor of Child Sexual Abuse, Counselling a Recovering Drug User, Counselling Young People, Counselling for Progressive Disability, Relationship Counselling: sons and their mothers, Responding to a Serious Mental Health Problem, Person-Centred Counselling Supervision: personal and professional, Counselling Victims of Warfare, Counselling for Eating Disorders in Men, Counselling for Obesity* and *Counselling for Problem Gambling.* The aim of the series is to bring the reader a direct experience of the counselling process, an exposure to the thoughts and feelings of both client and counsellor as they encounter each other on the therapeutic journey, and an insight into the value and importance of supervision.

Richard is also writing his first novel, 'Dying to Live', a story of traumatic loss, alcohol use and the therapeutic and has also adapted one of his books as a stage or radio play, and plans to do the same to other books in the series if the first is successful. However, he is currently seeking an opportunity for it to be recorded or staged.

Richard is keen to bring the experience of the therapeutic process, from the standpoint and application of the person-centred approach, to a wider audience.

He is convinced that the principles and attitudinal values of this approach and the emphasis it places on the therapeutic relationship are key to helping people create greater authenticity both in themselves and in their lives, leading to a fuller and more satisfying human experience. By writing fictional accounts to try and bring the therapeutic process alive, to help readers engage with the characters within the narrative – client, counsellor and supervisor – he hopes to take the reader on a journey into the counselling room. Whether we think of it as pulling back the curtains or opening a door, it is about enabling people to access what can and does occur within the therapeutic process.

Acknowledgements

I would like to thank Pat Seber and Janet Thomas, both of whom are counsellors in the NHS, who kindly read through the first draft of this book and provided many helpful comments on the two cases. I also wish to thank the many people who I have met over the years, or worked with in various capacities within the NHS, who have contributed to my experience of the challenges that staff face and their dedication to providing quality healthcare.

Finally, once again, my thanks to everyone at Radcliffe Publishing for their support for this on-going series of books.

Introduction

The NHS is a vast and complex organisation that encompasses an incredibly diverse range of professions. All staff members are required to interface daily with people from very different backgrounds and with very different roles. From junior nursing staff to consultants, from secretaries to business managers, from technicians to site and services managers, the NHS brings together people in a myriad of relationships with the purpose of providing a healthcare system that meets the needs of patients now and in the future.

The NHS has unique tensions. Perhaps the major one relates to the way in which most NHS employees undertake their work out of a sense of vocation, from a sense of wanting to help others and to alleviate suffering and to cure the sick. Many NHS employees could obtain higher salaries in the private sector. But they choose to stay because there is something about being part of the NHS, something about working for an organisation founded on the principle of offering free healthcare to all.

The emotional and physical tolls of being confronted with the emotions of patients and relatives can become overwhelming. National health service staff members are expected to cope and maintain a professional service to patients at all times. But NHS staff members are human. What is 'soaked up' by them can get played out in group dynamics within teams, or in the family. To understand the intensity of these kinds of processes it is important to understand the NHS as a system, an interactive, some might say, 'living system'. Stress in any one area impacts on surrounding areas and can induce critical states in which distress, despair and frustration can no longer be contained. National health service staff members need space in which to 'let go'. This can occur through line-management, through supervision and sometimes within peer-support groups, but there can be times when a member of staff simply needs space away from managers, supervisors and anyone else in the team, to talk about how they are feeling, to release their pent-up feelings of sadness, frustration; whatever it is that has become too much to bear. And they will need to be able to feed back their experience so that the risk of future build-ups of pressure in the system can be minimised or avoided altogether.

The NHS is also a multi-cultural employer, with staff from probably every black minority ethnic group. It is a melting-pot of ethnic diversity within the UK. This brings challenges, yet also opportunities, for people to break down barriers and work together towards a common goal, drawing on individual's talents and skills to achieve a successful outcome.

Against this background, the need for suitable and appropriate staff support systems is critical, and in recent years the provision of staff counselling is an important element in ensuring that staff are psychologically and emotionally fit to play their part in the NHS.

Counselling in the NHS

Workplace counselling in the NHS has grown in scope over the last few decades, with many different areas of concern deserving of focus, and a growing number of published surveys and research papers. In 1998 Leeds and Sheffield universities conducted a large-scale study into stress in the NHS that demonstrated a link between stress and sickness absence (Borrill *et al.*, 1998). The Royal College of Nursing in its report *Counselling for Staff in Health Service Settings: a guide for employers and managers* cites its 'Working Well' survey of 6000 members saying 'staff experiencing significant levels of psychological distress report twice the mean level of shifts taken off sick than other colleagues' (RCN, 2002, p. 2).

Coles (2003, p. 31) draws on the experience of the North Staffordshire Combined NHS Healthcare Trust Staff Counselling Service, which was established in 1994. He lists the main work-related presentations as:

- work stress
- disciplinary matters
- harassment
- work relationships
- depression/anxiety (diagnosed by GP)
- lack of support/resources
- organisational change
- complaints
- violence/aggression.

However, the figures from the service also show that 'the majority of employees attending presented with personal problems', which Coles lists as follows:

- health problems
- personal relationship problems
- bereavement and loss
- domestic violence/aggression
- family problems
- alcohol
- sexual abuse
- depression/anxiety (diagnosed by GP) (Coles, 2003, p. 32).

An important question in the counselling of NHS staff is what is appropriate for an NHS staff counsellor to work with, given such a wide range of presenting problems? It is more a perceived difficulty, perhaps originating from the fact that we try to differentiate between problems based on what may be a false view that a particular issue can be treated in isolation – perhaps a reflection of the way in which medical models indicate a specific treatment for a particular condition. The difficulty is that psychological problems are not specific, and overlap. Stress at work and stress at home may be arising from two different sets of causes, but the symptoms experienced and presenting are likely to be the same. What, then, is the role of the NHS staff counsellor?

The Department of Health recommends three approaches to workplace counselling (DOH, 2000, pp. 7–8).

1 *Provision of face-to-face counselling*, within the framework of a 'short-term model of consultation' (i.e. approximately five to eight sessions).
2 *Telephone counselling*, allowing for self-referral and allowing clients choice as to whether to take it further is sometimes appropriate. (This should not be seen as an alternative to face-to-face contact but as a 'second means of accessing help'.)
3 *Response to traumatic incidents*, involving defusing, debriefing and post-trauma counselling.

It is interesting, as a counsellor, to read the language of this guidance as it refers to consultation – very much a medical view. However, and particularly from a person-centred perspective, clients do not consult their counsellor. It is much more of a relationship-based process with the very act of meeting up becoming and being the therapeutic process. Whilst there are, of course, specific issues to be dealt with, the counselling process is likely to extend beyond the presenting issues. This then raises the question of how far should this go, and whether time limited working is appropriate. I have discussed the matter of time limited counselling from a person-centred perspective elsewhere (Bryant-Jefferies, 2003b).

Workplace counselling

This book aims to demonstrate the application of the person-centred approach (PCA) – a theoretical approach to counselling that has, at its heart, the power of the relational experience – in the context of staff counselling in the NHS. It is this relational experience that I believe to be at the core of effective therapy, contributing to the possibility of releasing the client to realise their greater potential for authentic living. The approach is widely used by counsellors working in the UK today. In a membership survey in 2001 by the British Association for Counselling and Psychotherapy, 35.6 per cent of those responding claimed to work to the person-centred approach, whilst 25.4 per cent identified themselves as psychodynamic practitioners. However, whatever the approach, it seems to me that the relationship is the key factor in contributing to a successful outcome – though this must remain a very subjective concept for who, other than the client, can really define what experience is to be taken as a measure of a successful outcome?

The reader who has not read other titles in the *Living Therapy* (Radcliffe Publishing) series may find it takes a while to adjust to the dialogue format. Many of the responses offered by the counsellors, Alec and Barbara, are reflections of what their respective clients, Merle and Gerald, have said. This is not to be read as conveying a simple repetition of the clients' words. Rather, the counsellor seeks to voice empathic responses, often with a sense of 'checking out' that they are hearing accurately what the clients are saying. The client says something; the counsellor then conveys what they have heard, what they sense the client as having sought to communicate to them, sometimes with the same words, sometimes with words that include a sense of what they feel is being communicated through the client's tone of voice, facial expression, or simply the relational atmosphere of the moment. The client is then enabled to confirm that they have been heard accurately, or correct the counsellor in their perception. The client may then explore more deeply what they have been saying or move on, in either case with a sense that they have been heard and warmly accepted. To draw this to the reader's attention, I have included some of the inner thoughts and feelings that are present within the individuals who form the narrative.

The sessions are a little compressed. It is also fair to say that clients will take different periods of time before choosing to disclose particular issues, and will also take varying lengths of time in working with their own process. This book is not intended to in any way indicate the length of time that may be needed to work with the kinds of issues that are being addressed. The counsellor needs to be open and flexible to the needs of the client. For some clients, the process would take a lot longer. But there are also clients who are ready to talk about difficult experiences almost immediately – sometimes not feeling that they have much choice in the matter, as their own organismic processes are already driving memories, feelings, thoughts and experiences to the surface and into daily awareness.

The client (Merle) in Part 1 is experiencing being a target for oppression and possibly racism in her relationship with her manager. She is also experiencing work-related stress, partly as a result of the demands of her job as a community psychiatric nurse within a community mental health team, and also linked to the work that her manager requires her to undertake. She has also suffered a recent bereavement that has reduced her external support system and made it more difficult for her to cope with what is happening in her team. She feels exhausted and low in spirits.

The second client (Gerald) is experiencing work-related stress due to under-resourcing and the stress of his work as a service manager in the Accident and Emergency Department of a large NHS hospital trust. Staff shortages have added to his problems, along with a recent serious untoward incident (SUI). Whilst he has a supportive manager, his working life has had an adverse effect on his home life. He has begun drinking more heavily at home and on the way home, and his relationships with his wife and children have become problematic. He is not sleeping well and feels exhausted.

Both these clients are evidencing symptoms of depression and anxiety. Not all the sessions are included in the second dialogue. The aim is to convey a flavour of issues that can arise within an NHS managerial context (though there will, of course, be many others that could arise) and how the person-centred counsellor might respond to them.

The early sessions in each of the two cases in this book do not include lengthy assessment. The counsellor seeks to work towards building the therapeutic relationship by allowing the client to communicate what is pressing for him or her, although some information has previously been exchanged over the telephone. Untimely assessment can cut across a person-centred way of working, which is rooted in a trust that the client will bring to sessions what material he or she feels a need and a readiness to address. It is also a fact that this approach is more concerned with building a therapeutic relationship with the person and allowing the presence of the therapeutic conditions to effect constructive personality change rather than the counsellor 'doing' something specific to alleviate a given set of symptoms or focusing solely on a specific problem.

Some clients will need more than, say, six or eight counselling sessions and the staff counselling service will need to be clear as to how it is to respond, particularly as clients may not always know, or be able to convey at the start, how deep-seated a problem is, or what other issues may be associated with it which could arise during the counselling process. Time may need to be spent discussing options for on-going counselling or other forms of support.

What this book does not attempt to include is post-traumatic work, specifically processes of de-briefing that may be offered following a serious incident that has had a significant psychological effect on the client. I have discussed trauma and the person-centred approach elsewhere in the context of working with victims of warfare (Bryant-Jefferies, 2005) and a wealth of material has been written on therapeutic processes to help people deal with trauma and the issues that can arise. It is important to note, however, that counsellors in an NHS workplace setting may be drawn more into this kind of work, and they may feel that they need to undergo specific training to extend their competence in that area. It should not, however, be assumed by an organisation that staff employed as counsellors are therefore appropriate to work with teams, for instance, who have been affected by a serious incident.

For the person-centred counsellor there will also be questions around the assumptions made regarding trauma, the expectations that people will be affected in predictable ways and will need to work through it in a certain way. The person-centred approach affirms the uniqueness of the individual. The way they react and deal with dangerous and disturbing situations will depend on many factors, and these need to be taken into account.

I am also very mindful of employee attitudes to the NHS itself. This is particularly so in the case of Gerald, the second client, as he explores at length in one session his feelings towards the NHS as an organisation. Some might argue whether or not this is a therapeutic focus. However, for the manager working in the NHS, the organisational tensions will be contributing to NHS workplace stress. There will be clients who will need to air their views about the NHS, and this is one of the arguments for a counselling service that has a degree of independence. Counsellors who themselves are employed by the NHS may themselves be experiencing similar frustrations. This makes accurate empathy for the client's experience more difficult and could tempt self-disclosures on the part of the counsellor that are more a response to *their* need, rather than therapeutically valuable for the client.

In the text there are references to 'Agenda for Change' and 'Improving Working Lives', and these are described as they arise. The NHS is a huge employer, an organisation with tensions, some of which are unique to a healthcare environment, but many of which have relevance to those that arise in other workplace settings.

All the characters in the book are fictitious and are not intended to bear resemblance to any particular person or persons.

Supervision

The supervision sessions are included to offer the reader insight into the nature of therapeutic supervision in the context of the counselling profession, a method of supervising that I term 'collaborative review'. For many trainee counsellors, the use of supervision can be something of a mystery, and it is hoped that this book will go a long way to unravelling this. In the sessions I seek to demonstrate the application of the supervisory relationship. My intention is to show how supervision of a counsellor is an important part of the process of enabling a client to work through issues that in this case relate to traumatic events linked to stress in the workplace.

Many professions do not recognise the need for some form of personal and process supervision, and often what is offered is line-management. However, counsellors are required to receive regular supervision in order to explore the dynamics of their relationship with the client, the impact of the work on the counsellor and on the client, to receive support, to encourage professional development of the counsellor and to provide an opportunity for an experienced co-professional to monitor the supervisee's work in relation to ethical standards and codes of practice. It is hoped that the supervision sessions will help readers from other professions to recognise the value of some form of collaborative support in order to help them become more authentically present with their clients.

Merry described what he termed as 'collaborative inquiry' as a 'form of research or inquiry in which two people (the supervisor and the counsellor) collaborate or co-operate in an effort to understand what is going on within the counselling relationship and within the counsellor'. He emphasised how this 'moves the emphasis away from "doing things right or wrong" (which seems to be the case in some approaches to supervision) to "how is the counsellor being, and how is that way of being contributing to the development of the counselling relationship based on the core conditions"' (Merry, 2002, p. 173). Elsewhere, Merry described the relationship between person-centred supervision and congruence, indicating that 'a state of congruence ... is the necessary condition for the therapist to experience empathic understanding and unconditional positive regard' (Merry, 2001, p. 183). Effective person-centred supervision provides a means through which congruence can be promoted within the therapist.

Tudor and Worrall (2004) have drawn together a number of theoretical and experiential strands from within and outside of the person-centred tradition in order to develop a position on the person-centred approach to supervision. They define the necessary factors for effective supervision within this way of working, and the respective responsibilities of both supervisor and supervisee in keeping with person-centred values and principles. They contrast person-centred working with other approaches to supervision and emphasise the importance of the therapeutic space as a place within which practitioners 'can dialogue freely between their personal philosophy and the philosophical assumptions which underlie their chosen theoretical orientation' (Tudor and Worrall, 2004, pp. 94–5). They affirm the values and attitudes of person-centred working and explore their application to the supervisory relationship.

It is the norm for all professionals working in the healthcare and social care environment in this age of regulation to be formally accredited or registered and to work to their own professional organisation's code of ethics or practice. For instance, registered counselling practitioners with the British Association for Counselling and Psychotherapy are required to have regular supervision and continuing professional development to maintain registration. Whilst professions other than counsellors will gain much from this book in their work, it is essential that they follow the standards, safeguards and ethical codes of their own professional organisation, and are appropriately trained and supervised to work with it on issues that arise. And in the context of the NHS, specific guidelines and policies of a particular organisation, with mindfulness of Health and Safety issues, must be followed.

The person-centred approach

The person-centred approach (PCA) was formulated by Carl Rogers, and references are made to his ideas within the text of this book. However, it will be helpful for readers who are unfamiliar with this way of working to have an appreciation of its theoretical base.

Rogers proposed that certain conditions, when present within a therapeutic relationship, would enable the client to develop towards what he termed 'fuller functionality'. Over a number of years he refined these ideas, which he defined as 'the necessary and sufficient conditions for constructive personality change'. These he described as follow.

1 Two persons are in psychological contact.
2 The first, whom we shall term the client, is in a state of incongruence, being vulnerable or anxious.

3 The second person, whom we shall term the therapist, is congruent or integrated in the relationship.
4 The therapist experiences unconditional positive regard for the client.
5 The therapist experiences an empathic understanding of the client's internal
   frame of reference and endeavours to communicate this experience to the
   client.
6 The communication to the client of the therapist's empathic understanding
   and unconditional positive regard is to a minimal degree achieved (Rogers,
   1957, p. 96).

The first necessary and sufficient condition given for constructive personality
change is that of 'two persons being in psychological contact'. However,
although Rogers later published this as simply 'contact' (Rogers, 1959) it is suggested (Wyatt and Sanders, 2002, p. 6) that this was actually written in 1953–4.
They quote Rogers as defining contact in the following terms: 'Two persons are in
psychological contact, or have the minimum essential relationship when each
makes a perceived or subceived difference in the experiential field of the other'
(Rogers, 1959, p. 207). A recent exploration of the nature of psychological contact from a person-centred perspective is given by Warner (2002).

Contact

There is much to reflect on when considering a definition of 'contact' or 'psychological contact'. Is it the case that contact is either present or not; or is it a continuum with greater or lesser degrees exhibited? It seems to me that it is both.
Rather like the way that light may be regarded as either a particle or a wave,
contact may be seen as a specific state of being, or as a process, depending upon
what the perceiver is seeking to measure or observe. If I am trying to observe or
measure whether there is contact, then my answer will be in terms of 'yes' or 'no'.
If I am seeking to determine the degree to which contact exists, then the answer
will be along a continuum. In other words, from the moment of minimal contact there is contact, but it can then extend as more aspects of the client become
present within the therapeutic relationship which, itself, may at times reach
moments of increasing depth.

Empathy

Rogers defined empathy as meaning 'entering the private perceptual world of the
other ... being sensitive, moment by moment, to the changing felt meanings
which flow in this other person ... It means sensing meanings of which he or
she is scarcely aware, but not trying to uncover totally unconscious feelings'
(Rogers, 1980, p. 142). It is a very delicate process, and it provides a foundation
block to effective person-centred therapy. The counsellor's role is primarily to

establish empathic rapport and communicate empathic understanding to the client. This latter point is vital. Empathic understanding only has therapeutic value where it is communicated to the client.

I would like to add another comment regarding empathy. There is so much more to it than simply letting the client know what you understand from what they have communicated. It is also, and perhaps more significantly, the actual *process* of listening to a client, of attending – facial expression, body language, and presence – that is being offered and communicated and received *at the time that the client is speaking, at the time that the client is experiencing what is present for them*. It is, for the client, the knowing that, in the moment of an experience the counsellor is present and striving to be an understanding companion.

Unconditional positive regard

Within the therapeutic relationship the counsellor seeks to maintain an attitude of unconditional positive regard towards the client and all that they disclose. This is not 'agreeing with', it is simply warm acceptance of the fact that the client is being how they need or choose to be. Rogers wrote, 'when the therapist is experiencing a positive, acceptant attitude towards whatever the client *is* at that moment, therapeutic movement or change is more likely to occur' (Rogers, 1980, p. 116). Mearns and Thorne suggest that 'unconditional positive regard is the label given to the fundamental attitude of the person-centred counsellor towards her client. The counsellor who holds this attitude deeply values the humanity of her client and is not deflected in that valuing by any particular client behaviours. The attitude manifests itself in the counsellor's consistent acceptance of and enduring warmth towards her client' (Mearns and Thorne, 1988, p. 59).

Wilkins and Bozarth assert that 'unconditional positive regard is the curative factor in person-centred therapy' (Bozarth and Wilkins, 2001, p. vii). It is perhaps worth speculatively drawing these two statements together. We might then suggest that the unconditional positive regard experienced and conveyed by the counsellor, and received by the client, as an expression of the counsellor's valuing of their client's humanity, has a curative role in the therapeutic process. We might then add that this may be the case more specifically for those individuals who have been affected by a lack of unconditional warmth and prizing in their lives.

Congruence

Last, but by no means least, is that state of being that Rogers referred to as congruence, but which has also been described in terms of 'realness', 'transparency', 'genuineness', 'authenticity'. Indeed Rogers wrote that '. . . genuineness, realness or congruence . . . this means that the therapist is openly being the feelings and attitudes that are flowing within at the moment . . . the term transparent catches the flavour of this condition' (Rogers, 1980, p. 115). Putting this into the therapeutic setting, we can say that 'congruence is the state of being of the counsellor when her outward responses to her client consistently match the inner feelings and sensations which she has in relation to her client' (Mearns and Thorne, 1999, p. 84). Interestingly, Rogers makes the following comment in his interview with Richard Evans that with regard to the three conditions; 'first, and most important, is therapist congruence or genuineness . . . one description of what it means to be congruent in a given moment is to be aware of what's going on in your experiencing at that moment, to be acceptant towards that experience, to be able to voice it if it's appropriate, and to express it in some behavioural way' (Evans, 1975).

I would suggest that any congruent expression by the counsellor of their feelings or reactions has to emerge through the process of being in therapeutic relationship with the client. Indeed, the condition indicates that the therapist is congruent or integrated into the relationship. This indicates the significance of the relationship. Being congruent is a disciplined way of being and not an open door to endless self-disclosure. Congruent expression is perhaps most appropriate and therapeutically valuable where it is informed by the existence of an empathic understanding of the client's inner world, and is offered in a climate of a genuine warm acceptance towards the client. Having said that, it is reasonable to suggest that, taking Rogers' comment quoted above that regarding congruence as 'most important' we might suggest that unless the therapist is congruent in themselves and in the relationship, then their empathy and unconditional positive regard would be at risk of not being authentic or genuine.

Another view, however, would be that it is in some way false to distinguish or rather seek to separate out the three 'core conditions', that they exist together as a whole, mutually dependent on the presence of the others in order to ensure that therapeutic relationship is established.

Perception

There is also the sixth condition, of which Rogers wrote: 'the final condition . . . is that the client perceives, to a minimal degree, the acceptance and empathy which the therapist experiences for him. Unless some communication of these attitudes has been achieved, then such attitudes do not exist in the relationship as far as the client is concerned, and the therapeutic process could not, by our hypothesis, be initiated' (Rogers, 1957). It is interesting that he uses the words 'minimal degree', suggesting that the client does not need to fully perceive the fullness of the empathy and unconditional positive regard present within, and communicated by, the counsellor. A glimpse accurately heard and empathically understood is enough to have positive, therapeutic effect although logically one might think that the more that is perceived, the greater the therapeutic impact. But if it is a matter of intensity and accuracy, then a client experiencing a vitally important fragment of their inner world being empathically understood may be more significant to them, and more therapeutically significant, than a great deal being heard less accurately and with a weaker sense of therapist understanding. The communication of the counsellors' empathy, congruence and unconditional positive regard, received by the client, creates the conditions for a process of constructive personality change.

Relationship is key

The PCA regards the relationship with clients, and the attitude held within that relationship, to be key factors. In my experience, many adult psychological difficulties develop out of life experiences that involve problematic, conditional or abusive relational experiences. This can be centred in childhood or later in life, and in this book we focus on the NHS. What is significant is that the individual is left, through relationships that have a negative conditioning effect, with a distorted perception of themselves and their potential as a person. Patterns are established in early life, bringing their own particular problems, however they can be exacerbated by conditional and psychologically damaging experiences later in life in the NHS workplace for example, that in some cases will have a resonance to what has occurred in the past, exacerbating the effects still further.

An oppressive experience in the NHS workplace can undermine a staff member's confidence; leaving them anxious, uncertain and moving towards establishing patterns of thought, feeling and behaviour associated with the developing concept of themselves, typified by 'I am weak and cannot expect to be treated any differently'; 'I just have to accept this attitude towards me, what can I do to change anything?'. These psychological conclusions may rest on patterns of thinking and feeling already established, perhaps the person was bullied at school, or experienced rejection in the home. They may have had a life time of stress, or it may be a relatively new experience, leading to a way of thinking developing typified by 'it's normal to feel stressed, you just keep going, whatever it takes' – until the day arrives when the person is so overloaded that they breakdown under the pressure, and may then require a significant length of time in order to recover, something that could have been avoided had the NHS workplace culture been different and opportunities made available *and accessible* to deal with the build-up of stress.

The result is a conditioned sense of self, with the individual thinking, feeling and acting in ways that enable them to maintain their self-beliefs and meanings within their learned or adapted concept of self. These are then lived out, the person seeking to satisfy what they have come to believe about themselves: needing to care either because it has been normalised, or in order to prove to themselves and the world that they are a 'good' person. They will need to maintain this conditioned sense of self and the sense of satisfaction that this gives them when it is lived out because they have developed such a strong identity with it.

The term 'conditions of worth' applies to the conditioning mentioned previously that is frequently present in childhood, and at other times in life, when a person experiences that their worth is conditional on their doing something, or behaving, in a certain way. This is usually to satisfy someone else's needs, and can be contrary to the client's own sense of what would be a satisfying experience. The values of others become a feature of the individual's structure of self. The person moves away from being true to themselves, learning instead to remain 'true' to their conditioned sense of worth. This state of being in the client is challenged by the person-centred therapist by offering them unconditional positive regard and warm acceptance. Such a therapist, by genuinely offering these therapeutic attitudes, provides the client with an opportunity to be exposed to what may be a new experience or one that in the past they have dismissed, preferring to stay with that which matches and therefore reinforces their conditioned sense of worth and sense of self.

By offering someone a non-judgemental, warm and accepting, and authentic relationship – (perhaps a kind of 'therapeutic love') – that person can grow into a fresh sense of self in which their potential as a person is more fulfilled. Such an experience fosters an opportunity for the client to redefine themselves as they experience the presence of the therapist's congruence, empathy and unconditional positive regard. This process can take time. Often the personality change that is required to sustain a shift away from what have been termed 'conditions of worth' may require a lengthy period of therapeutic work, bearing in mind that the person may be struggling to unravel a sense of self that has been developed, sustained and reinforced for many decades of life. Of course, where they have been established more recently, for instance in response to NHS workplace experience, then less time may be necessary.

Actualising tendency

A crucial feature or factor in this process of 'constructive personality change' is the presence of what Rogers termed 'the actualising tendency'; a tendency towards fuller and more complete personhood with an associated greater fulfilment of their potentialities. The role of the person-centred counsellor is to provide the facilitative climate within which this tendency can work constructively. The 'therapist trusts the actualizing tendency of the client and truly believes that the client who experiences the freedom of a fostering psychological climate will resolve his or her own problems' (Bozarth, 1998, p. 4). This is fundamental to the application of the person-centred approach. Rogers (1986, p. 198) wrote: 'the person-centred approach is built on a basic trust in the person ... [It] depends on the actualizing tendency present in every living organism – the tendency to grow, to develop, to realize its full potential. This way of being trusts the constructive directional flow of the human being towards a more complex and complete development. It is this directional flow that we aim to release.'

Having said the above, we must also acknowledge that for some people, or at certain stages, rather than producing a liberating experience, there will instead be a tendency to maintain the status quo, perhaps the fear of change, the uncertainty, or the implications of change are such that the person prefers to maintain the known, the certain. In a sense, there is a liberation from the imperative to change and grow which may bring temporary – and perhaps permanent – relief for the person. The actualising tendency may work through the part of the person that needs relief from change, enhancing its presence for the period of time that the person experiences a need to maintain this. The person-centred therapist will not try to move the person from this place or state. It is to be accepted, warmly and unconditionally. And, of course, sometimes in the moment of acceptance the person is enabled to question whether that really is how they want to be.

Configuration within self

It is of value to draw attention, at this point, to the notion of 'configurations within self'. Configurations within self (Mearns and Thorne, 2000) are discrete sets of thoughts, feelings and behaviours that develop through the experience of life. They emerge in response to a range of experiences including the process of introjection and the symbolisation of experiences, as well as in response to dissonant self-experience within the person's structure of self. They can also exist in what Mearns terms as 'growthful' and 'not for growth' configurations (Mearns and Thorne, 2000, pp. 114–6); each offering a focus for the actualising tendency, the former seeking an expansion into new areas of experience with all that that brings, the latter seeking to energise the status quo and to block change because of its potential for disrupting the current order within the structure of self. The actualising tendency may not always manifest through growth or developmental change. It can also manifest through periods of stabilisation and stability, or a wanting to get away from something – a retreat into sickness absence, perhaps, in the NHS context. In the counselling process, as the client gains fuller contact with his or her own experience and develops a greater sense of trust, the counsellor will be encouraged to voice and explore this, drawing it into the open, into awareness, from which it can more effectively be worked with.

Mearns suggests that these 'parts' or 'configurations' interrelate 'like a family, with an individual variety of dynamics'. As within any 'system', change in one area will impact on its functioning. He therefore comments that 'when the interrelationship of configurations changes, it is not that we are left with something entirely new: we have the same "parts" as before, but some which may have been subservient before are stronger, others which were judged adversely are accepted, some which were in self-negating conflict have come to respect each other, and overall the parts have achieved constructive integration with the energy release which arises from such fusion' (Mearns, 1999, pp. 147–8). The growing acceptance of the configurations, their own fluidity and movement within the self-structure, the increased, open and more accurate communication between the parts, is perhaps another way of considering the integrating of the threads of experience to which Rogers refers.

Understanding the configurational nature of ourselves enables us to understand why we are triggered into certain thoughts, feelings and behaviours, and how they group together, serving a particular experiential purpose for the person. From this theoretical perspective we can argue that the person-centred counsellor's role is essentially facilitative. Creating the therapeutic climate of empathic understanding, unconditional positive regard and authenticity creates a relational climate which encourages the client to move into a more fluid state with more openness to their own experience and the discovery of a capacity towards a fuller actualising of their potential.

Relationship re-emphasised

In addressing these factors the therapeutic relationship is central. A therapeutic approach such as person-centred affirms that it is not what you do so much as *how you are* with your client that is therapeutically significant, and this 'how you are' has to be received by the client. Gaylin (2001, p. 103) highlights the importance of client perception. 'If clients believe that their therapist is working on their behalf – if they perceive caring and understanding – then therapy is likely to be successful. It is the condition of attachment and the perception of connection that have the power to release the faltered actualization of the self.' He goes on to stress how 'we all need to feel connected, prized – loved', describing human beings as 'a species born into mutual interdependence, and that there 'can be no self outside the context of others. Loneliness is dehumanizing and isolation anathema to the human condition. The relationship,' he suggests 'is what psychotherapy is all about.'

Love is an important word though not necessarily one often used to describe therapeutic relationship. Patterson, however, gives a valuable definition of love as it applies to the person-centred therapeutic process. He writes, 'we define love as an attitude that is expressed through empathic understanding, respect and compassion, acceptance, and therapeutic genuineness, or honesty and openness towards others' (Patterson, 2000, p. 315). We all need love, but most of all we need it during our developmental period of life. The same author affirms that 'whilst love is important throughout life for the well-being of the individual, it is particularly important, indeed absolutely necessary, for the survival of the infant and for providing the basis for the normal psychological development of the individual' (Patterson, 2000, pp. 314–5). In a previous book in this series I used the analogy of treating a wilting plant (Bryant-Jefferies, 2003a, p. 12). We can spray it with some specific herbicide or pesticide to eradicate a perceived disease that may be present in that plant, and that may be enough. But perhaps the true cause of the disease is that the plant is located in harsh surroundings, perhaps too much sun and not enough water, poor soil, near other plants that it finds difficulty in surviving so close to. Maybe by offering the plant a healthier environment that will facilitate greater nourishment according to the needs of the plant, it may become the strong, healthy plant it has the potential to become. Yes, the chemical intervention may also be helpful, but if the true causes of the diseases are environmental – essentially the plant's relationship with that which surrounds it – then it won't actually achieve sustainable growth. We may not be able to transplant it, but we can provide water, nutrients and maybe shade it from a fierce sun. Therapy, it seems to me, exists to provide this healthy environment within which the 'wilting' client can begin the process of receiving the 'nourishment' (in the form of healthy relational experience) that can enable them, in time, to become a more fully functioning person.

Process of change from a person-centred perspective

Rogers was interested in understanding the process of change, what it was like, how it occurred and what experiences it brought to those involved – client and therapist. At different points he explored this. Embleton Tudor *et al.* (2004) point to a model consisting of 12 steps identified in 1942 (Rogers, 1942) and to his two later chapters on this topic (Rogers, 1951), and finally the seven-stage model in 1958/1967. He wrote of 'initially looking for elements which would mark or characterize change itself'. However, what he experienced from his enquiry and research into the process of change he summarised as: 'individuals move, I began to see, not from fixity or homeostasis through change to a new fixity, though such a process is indeed possible. But much the more significant continuum is from fixity to changingness, from rigid structure to flow, from stasis to process. I formed the tentative hypothesis that perhaps the qualities of the client's expression at any one point might indicate his position on this continuum, where he stood in the process of change' (Rogers, 1967a, p. 131).

   Change, then, involves a movement from fixity to greater fluidity, from, we might say, a rigid set of attitudes and behaviours to a greater openness to experience, to variety and diversity. Change might be seen as having a certain liberating quality, a freeing up of the human being – his heart, mind, emotions – so that the person experiences themselves less as a fixed object and more as a conscious process. The list below is taken from Rogers' summary of the process, indicating the changes that people will show.

1   This process involves a loosening of feelings.
2   This process involves a change in the manner of experiencing.
3   The process involves a shift from incongruence to congruence.
4   The process involves a change in the manner in which, and the extent to which the individual is able and willing to communicate himself in a receptive climate.
5   The process involves a loosening of the cognitive maps of experience.
6   There is a change in the individual's relationship to his problem.
7   There is a change in the individual's manner of relating (Rogers, 1967a, pp. 156–8).

This is a brief overview; the chapter in which he describes the process of change has much more detail and should be read in order to gain a clear grasp not only of the process as a whole, but of the distinctive features of each stage, as he saw it. Embleton Tudor *et al.* summarise this process in the following, and I think helpful, terms: 'a movement from fixity to fluidity, from closed to open, from tight to loose, and from afraid to accepting' (Embleton Tudor *et al.*, 2004, p. 47).

In Rogers' description of the process he makes the point that there were several types of process in which personality changes, and that the process he described is one that is 'set in motion when the individual experiences himself as being fully received'. Does this process apply to all psychotherapies? Rogers indicated that more data were needed, adding that 'perhaps therapeutic approaches which place great stress on the cognitive and little on the emotional aspects of experience may set in motion an entirely different process of change'. In terms of whether this process of change would generally be viewed as desirable and that it would move the person in a valued direction, Rogers expressed the view that the valuing of a particular process of change was linked to social value judgements made by individuals and cultures. He pointed out that the process of change that he described could be avoided, simply by people 'reducing or avoiding those relationships in which the individual is fully received as he is'.

Rogers also took the view that change was unlikely to be rapid, making the point that many clients enter the therapeutic process at stage two, and leave at stage four, having during that period gained enough to feel satisfied. He suggested it would be 'very rare, if ever, that a client who fully exemplified stage one would move to a point where he fully exemplified stage seven', and that if this did occur 'it would involve a matter of years' (Rogers, 1967a, pp. 155–6). He wrote of how, at the outset, the threads of experience are discerned and understood separately by the client but as the process of change takes place, they move into 'the flowing peak moments of therapy in which all these threads become inseparably woven together.' He continues, 'in the new experiencing with immediacy which occurs at such moments, feeling and cognition interpenetrate, self is subjectively present in the experience, volition is simply the subjective following of a harmonious balance of organismic direction. Thus, as the process reaches this point the person becomes a unity of flow, of motion. He has changed, but what seems most significant, he has become an integrated process of changingness' (Rogers, 1967a, p. 158).

It conjures up images of flowing movement, perhaps we should say purposeful flowing movement, as being the essence of the human condition, a state that we each have the potential to become, or to realise. Is it something we generate or develop out of fixity, or does it exist within us all as a potential that we lose during our conditional experiencing in childhood or later in life? Are we discovering something new, or re-discovering something that was lost?

I am extremely encouraged by the increasing interest in the PCA, the growing amount of material being published, and the realisation that relationship is a key factor in positive therapeutic outcome. There is currently much debate about theoretical developments within the person-centred world and its application. Discussions on the theme of Rogers' therapeutic conditions presented by various key members of the person-centred community have been published (Bozarth and Wilkins, 2001; Haugh and Merry, 2001; Wyatt, 2001; Wyatt and Sanders,

2002). Mearns and Thorne have produced a timely publication revising and developing key aspects of person-centred theory (Mearns and Thorne, 2000). Wilkins has produced a book that addresses most effectively many of the criticisms levelled against person-centred working (Wilkins, 2003) and Embleton Tudor *et al.* (2004) have written an introduction to the person-centred approach that places the theory and practice within a contemporary context. Recently, Howard Kirschenbaum (Carl Rogers' biographer) published an article entitled 'The current status of Carl Rogers and the person-centered approach'. In his research for this article he noted that from 1946–86, 84 books, 64 chapters, and 456 journal articles were published on Carl Rogers and the person-centred approach. In contrast, from 1987–2004 141 books, 174 book chapters and 462 journal articles were published. A clear trend towards more publications and, presumably, more readership and interest in the approach. Also, he noted that there are now some 50 person-centred publications available around the world, mostly journals, and there are now person-centred organisations in 18 countries, and 20 organisations overall. He also draws attention to the large body of research demonstrating the effectiveness of person-centred therapy, concluding that the person-centred approach is 'alive and well' and appears to be experiencing 'something of a revival, both in professional activity and academic respectability' (Kirschenbaum, 2005). There are many other books, and perhaps there is a need now for a comprehensive database of all person- or client-centred books to be made available to all training organisations and person-centred networks. And perhaps it already exists.

Person-centred theory affirms the importance of congruence, of being genuine, authentic, transparent, and at a time when the world seems to be embracing quite the opposite. It seems to me that the relational component of the person-centred approach, based on the presence of the core conditions, is emerging strongly as a counter to the sense of isolation that frequently accompanies deep psychological and emotional problems, and which is a feature of materialistic societies. It is fascinating that this is occurring now given that the concept of relational counselling was very much a driving force in the early development of the ideas that then developed into what we know as the person-centred approach.

Of the counselling relationship Rogers wrote in 1942: 'The counselling relationship is one in which warmth of acceptance and absence of any coercion or personal pressure on the part of the counsellor permits the maximum expression of feelings, attitudes, and problems by the counsellee . . . In the unique experience of complete emotional freedom within a well-defined framework the client is free to recognize and understand his impulses and patterns, positive and negative, as in no other relationship' (Rogers, 1942, pp. 113–14).

This is obviously a very brief introduction to the approach. Person-centred theory continues to develop as practitioners and theoreticians consider its application in various fields of therapeutic work and extend our theoretical understanding of developmental and therapeutic processes. At times it feels like it has become more than just individuals, rather it feels like a group of colleagues, based around the world, working together to penetrate deeper towards a more complete theory of the human condition, and this includes people from the many traditions and schools of thought. Person-centred or client-centred theory and practice has a key role in this process. Theories are being revisited and developed, new ideas speculated upon, new media explored for presenting the core values and philosophy of the person-centred approach. It is an exciting time.

PART I

The oppressed nurse

CHAPTER 1

Counselling session 1: disclosing a bereavement and an unsupportive manager

It was a miserable day, cold and wet, and Merle sat in the waiting area wondering to herself whether she was doing the right thing. She felt she needed to talk to someone, work had become a real struggle. Her work in the Community Mental Health Team was stressful and demanding, and there often seemed to be staff shortages, but that wasn't what had caused her to make contact with the staff counselling service at the NHS Trust. It had been the death of her aunt. Although it had happened some months ago now, somehow it had only been later that she had come to realise just how much she missed her. She had always been the person she had turned to for advice. They had been close for many years.

It wasn't that she wasn't close to her mother, but, well, her mother had her own problems, she was often depressed, and from an early age Merle had naturally gravitated towards her aunt Sarah. Now her aunt had died and Merle found herself feeling quite alone. She knew that she wasn't, she had friends, and her brother although she never really got on that well with him. No, everything had become more of a struggle, particularly at work where the demands had become unmanageable. She was not alone in feeling this, but she felt that she, in particular, carried the highest caseload of the most difficult and demanding patients.

She glanced at her watch. She could feel her anxiety rising as she noted that it was almost 10.30 am, the time for her appointment. She wondered whether she had time to leave, just forget about it and get on with it as best she could. But the truth was she knew she couldn't. She was struggling to hold herself together. She had to talk, had to. She felt so empty inside, and so weak. She didn't like it. It didn't come naturally to her. She was used to working hard, being organised, knowing what she was doing and doing a good job.

But her boss had been on at her again, she felt singled out. And he didn't seem to take into account how she was feeling after her aunt's death. He'd somewhat grudgingly agreed to her having time off for the funeral, muttering how it was going to upset the rota with so many people on holiday.

As she sat lost in her own thoughts she didn't hear her name being called. It was only when it was spoken again that she realised someone was standing in front of her, and she brought herself out of her thoughts.

'Hello. You must be Merle. I'm Alec, one of the counsellors. We spoke on the phone.'

'Hello, yes.' She stood up. Alec was smiling. He looked quite relaxed.

'The room's along the corridor. Can I get you tea or coffee?'

'Er, no, no thanks. I'll be fine.'

'Sure?'

'Yes, thanks.'

Merle walked into the counselling room and turned to ask where to sit.

'Whichever, up to you.'

Merle chose the seat closest to the door, she wasn't sure why, maybe force of habit. As a community psychiatric nurse she often sat closest to the door with clients in case there was a problem and she needed to get out. Not that she felt there might be a problem, it was just something she did, pretty much without thinking.

Alec asked if there was anything Merle wanted to ask about the counselling. He had already talked to her on the phone about confidentiality and the fact that there was a limit of eight sessions, and in particular that although he came under the Human Resources Department, he was in fact separate and was not there to pass information on to anyone. Also, he had made it clear that the actual counselling service was offered in a different building, with its own room and waiting area to try and ensure greater confidentiality. Although he was employed by the Trust, the counselling team operated as an independent unit.

Merle had felt reassured by this, she wasn't sure whether having counselling was something that would count against her when she sought promotion. She had thought not, but she also knew that in the NHS confidentiality wasn't always as tight as it could be. She had realised how different people had different meanings for confidentiality when a counsellor had joined their Community Mental Health Team (CMHT). At first she had thought she was being rather precious, not wanting to say much about the content of sessions, but gradually she began to understand that there were going to be topics that a client would want to talk about and which they may not want to disclose to their key worker. Of course, there was agreement in the team that anything disclosed that was significant in relation to a patient's treatment would be shared, but generally with the patient's agreement, and then only specific information.

'So, we have eight sessions of counselling, and you can use as many of those sessions as you like. I hope by listening and giving you space and time to talk you can resolve the difficulties that you are encountering.' Alec knew from the phone call that Merle's aunt's death had been the main cause of her referring, but he was also aware as well that she had mentioned work getting on top of her. He didn't know which area Merle would want to focus on and in line with his person-centred approach he was not going to direct her one way or the other. He trusted that Merle would know for herself what was most pressing, or what she felt she needed, or felt most able, to talk about.

In a time limited setting there can be an underlying agenda to enable an employee to get well so they can get back to work, or get back to working as effectively and efficiently as they have in the past. However, this may not be the issue most on a client's mind, and it is important, if a genuinely person-centred approach is to be offered, that the client is given the freedom to choose. The client knows that the counselling is being offered in an NHS context and therefore there is an NHS agenda. But the counsellor will not want to reinforce that.

This is an issue for NHS staff counselling as very often a client is assessed, possibly by someone other than the counsellor who will work with the client, and a treatment plan will be devised which the counsellor will be required to work to. This can be counter-productive, limiting the client to particular issues and cutting across the possibility of a more holistic counselling process. Presenting issues may not always be the root cause of problems or difficulties. However, at the same time it has to be acknowledged that we live and work in a world that is extremely sensitive to the question of *risk*. Employers have responsibilities for ensuring they are not contributing to risk among their staff. Risk assessment has become an increasingly recognised feature of assessment and it is likely to remain this way.

The person-centred counsellor would be likely to be responding with questions as to who is feeling at risk – organisation, employee, counsellor – and who defines risk? At the same time, concern about a client's well-being can be seen as an expression of positive regard, of warmth. The danger is that what becomes conveyed is just that, positive regard attached to a hope that risks will diminish rather than genuine unconditional positive regard for a client who, from their standpoint, needs to maintain the presence of risk as part of their way of being, and who might need to talk about what risk means to them without feeling that a counsellor is in some way pressuring or urging them to change.

With regard to general assessment, the argument can be made that without sufficient direction and focus the client won't address what they need to. From a person-centred perspective the client should be trusted to know what they need to do. The client's internal locus of evaluation should be respected. They know where they are hurting, where they are feeling under stress, and they know that they want to feel better. The person-centred counsellor wants to create a therapeutic relationship in which the client can bring as much, or as little, of themselves as they wish, trusting that the client will make as much use of the counselling opportunity as they can. The client needs to work at their own pace. Pushing a client along is not necessarily helpful, and is certainly outside of person-centred practice. And if not enough work has been done perhaps the client simply needs more time.

'I guess I'm here because, well, I don't feel I'm coping too well.' She lapsed into silence. 'I can't seem to concentrate, I get irritable, I don't sleep too well and, I don't know, I just feel so tired, you know?'

Alec nodded, 'so a lot of things that are uncomfortable'. Alec deliberately didn't repeat them all back. He wasn't a member of the reflection school of empathy. And besides, he didn't want some listening technique to get in the way. Merle was clearly uncomfortable by all these things, he wanted to acknowledge that and leave her free to choose which she wanted to talk about.

'Yeah, really uncomfortable, you know? Like, it's not me, yeah?'

'Mhmm, not you.'

'Things get me down and, well, I've always coped, yeah, always kept my head down and got on with stuff. I really did.' She shook and lowered her head. 'Now I just wish my aunt was around to talk to.' She looked up, 'no disrespect to you, but . . .'

'Yes, yes, I know, it's not the same and it can never be the same.'

Merle bit her lip as she felt her eyes watering. She opened her bag and took out a tissue, dabbing at the underside of her eye and trying not to disturb her make up.

'They say it won't run but, well, that's what they say . . .' She smiled, bringing herself away a little from the upset she felt for the loss of her aunt.

'Yes.'

Merle was aware of Alec's white skin, he seemed particularly pale, though she had noticed that with white men who had gingery-coloured hair. She wondered whether it might be different if he had a black skin like her, or if he had been a woman. Or would he be like her boss? She didn't think so, he already seemed to be listening to her, which was more than she felt at work. The thought lingered for a moment or two, and then passed.

'So, think I've lost my thread a bit here.'

'Well, it's not easy, you know, so take your time. You'd been saying about wishing your aunt was around to talk to, but you may have moved on from that now.'

Merle tightened her lips and lowered her face again. 'No, no, that's what's affected me.'

'And she was obviously someone special.' Alec deliberately did not add anything further.

This is a place when a counsellor might say something in reference to what the client might have talked about, for instance something like, 'You miss talking about the things that matter to you.' But that would be immediately directing the client towards the content of her conversations with her aunt and away from the simple fact of the client wishing her aunt was there. It may seem a small thing, but it is indicative of person-centred practice being very much a non-directive approach to counselling and psychotherapy.

'She was, she would listen, just listen, and she was so wise. She'd just calm me down. Just being with her. Sometimes just knowing she was there ...' Merle could feel the emotions rising within her and she couldn't finish the sentence.

'She offered so much.' Alec was aware straight away that perhaps his response was weak, that it was maybe too general and could more usefully have been a response to Merle's knowing that her aunt was there. But the moment had passed and Merle was responding to what he had said.

Merle nodded through her tears as she held the tissue to her face.

'I-miss-her-so-much.'

Alec was aware of the temptation to say something like, 'I know'. But he knew he didn't, not really. He stayed with his empathy, 'Yes, you miss her so much.'

Alec's response kept Merle centred in her feelings. She felt bereft, alone, and as if a huge part of herself was missing. Everything seemed too big, too much to cope with. She felt small, isolated, tired. Everything had become such an effort. Her feelings of sadness were very present for her as she continued to sit, continuing to hold the tissue to her face, sobbing and so wishing her aunt was still alive.

Time passed in silence. Merle sat, feeling a little spaced out in her head. The sobbing had stopped. 'Oh dear.' She took a deep breath. 'What am I going to do?'

Alec was unsure quite what Merle was referring to, though his initial assumption was that she was talking about coping with her feelings.

'What are you going to do about ...?' He left the question unanswered, seeking clarity so that he could more accurately empathise with what Merle was feeling.

'Work. I don't feel like I want to keep struggling on, not at the moment. I really don't. I used to love my work, I really did. Now ...' She shook her head. 'Now ...' She shrugged.

'Now it's different?' Again, a questioning tone as Alec sought to empathise and clarify what was happening for Merle.

She nodded. 'This is confidential, isn't it?'

'Yes. It's something about work?' He knew that Merle hadn't said this, but he felt it to be so and felt it would communicate his own empathic sensitivity to Merle's dilemma.

'I don't go round bad-mouthing people, that's not me, you know?'

'Sure, you're not someone that talks that way about people.'

Merle turned her head towards the window, watching, but not seeing, the raindrops falling on the window. She felt the tears welling up again in her own eyes. 'It's the team manager, he just makes me feel so small, so useless.'

'Mhmm, the way he behaves towards you, leaves you feeling small and useless.' Alec didn't say anything more, again keeping the focus on the feelings that Merle had described.

Merle felt herself not wanting to say anything more. She didn't like how she felt, she didn't want to feel that way. She hated it. But she felt as though she had no energy to fight it. Maybe she was being stupid, maybe she was imagining it all. She was just another black nurse, after all, to be hired and fired, at least, that's how it felt to her sometimes, particularly from some of the white managers, like her's. Didn't matter how hard she worked, she never got the credit, never got thanks for it, just given more to do. What was the point in fighting it? What was the point? Her aunt had told her, so many times, that was how it was. That was the way it worked. You had to keep your head down and get on with it. That one day it would work out, that it would be OK, she had to have faith. Truth was that whilst Merle believed what her aunt had said, she also didn't want to believe it either. Oh she didn't know, it was too much, too confusing, too complicated.

Merle continued to sit, staring down. Small and useless, the words stayed with her and she hated them the longer she dwelt on them. She didn't want to be that way. She thought back. It hadn't always been like that, far from it. And she'd always had so much enthusiasm for her work, but the last eighteen months were what seemed most real now, and it was during that time that her current boss had been in post. Was it all down to him, or was she really not as good a psychiatric nurse as she had thought. Maybe she wasn't. Maybe she was just distorting things and the truth was she wasn't good enough, couldn't handle the pressure. She didn't know. She just didn't know what to think.

Alec sat in the silence maintaining his attention on Merle as she sat. She seemed to look quite miserable, well, downcast was the word in his mind. Those last words had clearly been significant for her and it seemed to him that they remained very much in the room, hanging in the air, so to speak. They had clearly emerged from some place within Merle that was highly significant for her self-concept.

As he continued to sit in the silence he wondered whether he should say something further. It didn't feel uncomfortable in the sense of the actual silence feeling awkward, it actually felt as though Merle had connected with a significant part of herself and was being held there. He believed that when this was the case the client's own process needed to be trusted. Not that it shouldn't be trusted at all times, but in silences there was a process taking place and he would respect that. If Merle was dwelling on what had just been said then perhaps, in this moment, that is precisely what she needed to do. His role was to be a companion with her in that place. So anything he might say would be to affirm his presence. However, he didn't want to disturb her process or pull her out of the silence by reminding her of his presence. Indeed, it would be highly unlikely that she was unaware of him being there.

He noticed Merle take a deep breath and sigh. He wondered what had triggered that. He decided to acknowledge it. 'Makes you sigh.'

Empathy towards a particular behaviour can prove helpful. It communicates attention and offers opportunity for a client to say more about something if she wishes to. But the person-centred counsellor would not respond with something like, 'I wonder what that sigh means' which would have the effect of directing the client into thinking they have to explain their sigh. It may mean something, it may mean nothing. In this dialogue the counsellor simply notes it, communicates his attention, and leaves it at that.

Merle heard Alec speak. Yes, it does, she thought to herself.

'I just feel I am always having to prove myself, you know, have to be the best just to be good enough.' She was a little surprised by what she had said. Not that it was a new idea to her, but it was the way she said it, and the way that she felt. She was tired, tired of having to keep trying so much, and never getting any appreciation or thanks, just more work or some small matter that 'could be better', as she was often being told. 'He's, oh, look, I don't mean any disrespect to you, but he's white, and well, I think that's part of it. I'm the only black nurse in the team and I do feel singled out. He's not like he is with me with other people, I'm sure about it. Even some of the other staff members have said that they think I seem to get a hard time. Others, well, they don't seem to notice, or care. So, like I say, I don't seem to ever be able to be good enough, and I just feel I get treated unfairly. There's so much to do, I seem to get all the complex cases.' Merle felt desperate and tearful once again.

'Whatever you do doesn't meet your team manager's approval, and it really feels like it's to do with the way he reacts to your colour?' Alec could feel himself gritting his teeth, he didn't like racism. He pushed his reaction aside and sought to ensure he was maintaining his warmth and openness to Merle and what she needed to say and how she needed to be.

Merle nodded. Yes, she thought, he's the one. 'It doesn't matter how hard I try, it really doesn't. I just feel, like, what's the point?'

'Mhmm, like it's all too much and what is the point?' Alec was aware he had introduced the first part of his response, but it was very much the tone of what Merle was saying. He wanted to reflect in his empathy the impact on Merle of what she was saying as well as the words she was using.

Empathy is, of course, so much more than repeating back the words that a client has spoken. It is an attempt to convey what the counsellor understands from what the client is communicating, by using not only words but also tone of voice, mood, body language and the general atmosphere that what is being presented has generated. At the same time, the person-centred counsellor must be careful to own his or her reactions to what is being said, carefully distinguishing those rather than including them in such a way that they intrude on the client's sense of being heard.

If we take the notion of empathy as being the counsellor moving around within the client's inner world, then what he or she says must clearly be either what is being seen in that inner world in response to what the client is pointing out, or what the counsellor is experiencing in response to what has been pointed out. There will also be times when the counsellor may indicate what he or she senses to be present within that inner world and when this is introduced it should be done tentatively and certainly, not in any sense authoritatively.

'I'd feel better talking to my aunt, I know I would.' Merle felt a sudden rush of emotion once again as her attention turned back to her aunt Jessie. She was always so kind, so calming. She just had that way about her. Reassured her, yes, reassured her. That was what she did most. It would be OK. But now, well now it didn't feel OK, it didn't feel OK at all. But she didn't know what to do. It took her back to feeling small, powerless, she just wanted to go home and hide under the duvet cover, that was the truth of it.

She heard Alec's response, 'if only you could talk to your aunt, you know you'd feel better.'

Her thoughts were still with being under the duvet. As she thought about this her mother came to mind. She realised how that was what her mother did, and had done for years. Was she becoming like her mother? She really didn't want that. She thought of her father. He had stayed with them until she and her brother had left school, and then he'd left. She hadn't seen him for a while now. He'd always been a bit distant. Never said a lot at home. But then she'd spent a lot of her time with her aunt anyway as a child. Sitting in her front room on the orange sofa, drinking lemonade – she always made her own and it was, well, different, special, had a kind of bite to it that wasn't all sweet and sickly like the stuff in the cans. And cake, she made such wonderful cake. They only ever had supermarket cake at home.

Alec again did not disturb the silence that had emerged. He trusted that perhaps in the quiet of the counselling room there was time and space for Merle to maybe re-order her thoughts. He appreciated how, out in the world, so many different demands could invade a person's thinking, all the 'I should be doing this', or 'I ought to be doing that' which can take up so much of a person's thought life. We could spend so much time worrying about what we should be doing that we end up in a sense losing the present. So much human thought is taken up with worrying about the future or feeling perhaps bad about something in the past that was rather negative. There could be positives as well, but it can so take us away from engaging with the present.

He had noted a slight smile on Merle's face and wondered what had put it there. Should he respond – it was a contrast to the expression that had been there, and so whilst she was clearly very much in her own thoughts, there was something being communicated to him, albeit perhaps unconsciously.

Should empathy only be towards what the client is consciously communicating? If we take the holistic view then we must accept that as people we are often communicating information that we are unaware of. The counsellor must decide what to respond to. Or perhaps, rather than consider each piece of information he or she needs to be consistent in how much they respond, say, to facial expression or body language. At the same time, the stage of counselling may need to be considered. Too much empathy towards body language early on in a counselling relationship could feel quite threatening and invasive; the client feeling over-observed, as if their every movement is being analysed in some way. It's not that a person-centred counsellor will be analysing, that isn't their way of working, but the client may interpret it in that way and feel oppressed by it. This may be even more the case for a client for whom the issue of feeling oppressed is part of what they are bringing into counselling.

Having said that, a client may value the fact that someone has been attentive enough to recognise, say, a change of facial expression. The meaning they ascribe to that will vary from client to client, and may well be based on their past experience. A counsellor may be seen and experienced as overly attentive in the client's frame of reference and his or her empathy be interpreted as a kind of 'flirting'. Finding the most therapeutically helpful 'level' of empathy is part of the process of building a therapeutic relationship.

In this case we have a client feeling oppressed and undermined by her team manager. She is starting to explore this with her counsellor. The empathy shown by the counsellor must not oppress her, yet must be supportive and offer her a sense of feeling contained, feeling able to move around freely within herself and to be able to openly express what she experiences, and what comes into her awareness.

Interesting, Alec thought to himself, but I haven't really voiced much response to other facial expressions. Why just pick that out? He let the thought go after acknowledging it. He noticed the smile had changed back to what he perceived to be an expression of sadness. He decided to acknowledge this.

'I'm aware that your facial expression seemed to change to a smile and then back to what seems like sadness.'

Merle heard Alec's voice. She was feeling sad again. Another sigh. 'My aunt. I know I miss her, but maybe I miss her more than I thought.'

'Mhmm, more than you had appreciated.' He didn't use the same words, he knew how sometimes mirrored empathy could be irritating for a client, particularly in a first session when they are still adjusting to a counselling style of dialogue.

'Strange, but I feel a little calmer inside at the moment. The feelings are there, but somehow I feel different.'

'Mhmm, calmer, different in some way.' Alec kept the focus, this time using Merle's words. That was how it was with counselling. One minute you respond in one way, the next you respond in a manner that might be contradicting your previous rationale. But it was about being sensitive and responsive, being fluid, being able to distinguish where the client's words are important and need to be held, and where alternatives are appropriate.

Merle glanced up and noticed that time had passed, and that there were about ten minutes left of the session. Alec noticed the glance and responded, 'yes, about ten minutes left. I do want to check whether the way I am working with you, responding to you, is helpful and whether you want to continue, but I also don't want to take the focus away from what you have just said.'

'I think it is helpful. I mean, there aren't any answers, are there?'

'To?'

'To how I'm feeling. I mean, it's normal to feel sad when someone close dies, isn't it?'

Alec nodded. 'Yes.'

'It's just that, well, it feels more than that, you know, with work. And I realise I haven't said much about what I do, though I expect you've heard lots of other people and I don't suppose I'm much different.'

'Well, I have heard other people talk of their jobs, but everyone is different, everyone sees and reacts to their job differently.'

Merle sighed again. 'Yeah, I guess so. At the moment the thought of work just makes me want to hide, you know. I really don't know that I want to be there, not with how it is.'

'Mhmm, that sounds very clear, the way you have been affected leaves you feeling you just want to hide away and not be there.'

'But I can't do that. I have to keep going.'

Alec noted his temptation to say 'no, you have choices', but he also wanted to respect Merle's own view. 'You feel that you have to keep going.'

She nodded. 'Yeah, I'll be OK. I'll cope.'

'Mhmm, that sounds important for you to say that.'

Merle nodded. 'Yeah, well, you do, don't you?'

Alec sensed that Merle was in many ways probably preparing herself now to go back out into work, into her life beyond the counselling room. She'd allowed herself to engage with feelings – quite powerful feelings – during the session but was now in a sense re-affirming to herself how she needed to be. It was not unusual.

'I guess so. And I want to just say that you've engaged with a lot of feelings here, and it's an intense experience. So just ease yourself back into your routines, it can leave people feeling quite sensitive. I'm not saying that's how it will be for you, but it can be like that. Take care of yourself, yes?'

'Sure. So, when do I see you again?'

'When would be helpful and convenient?'

Merle hesitated. 'Now I've started I'd like to come weekly. I do still feel a bit calmer, you know, and I like that.' She paused, biting her lip.

'Something wrong?'

'Well, I'm on a day's leave today – didn't want to tell my boss I was coming to counselling.'

'You're entitled to come to counselling in work time.'

'I know, but, well, I just think it won't go down too well.'

This is a difficult issue. A client is entitled to seek counselling support, and in work time, but, the manager would expect to know when a client is away from their desk. So a balance has to be struck. This, however, is particularly difficult in this kind of situation where the behaviour of the manager is a major factor in counselling being sought. The staff member might say that they have an appointment with Human Resources, but he could phone to check it out and be told no, because they are not necessarily going to be aware of who is being seen for counselling.

Employers have a responsibility to ensure that there is a clear understanding among managers of the rights of staff to attend counselling, and that a suitable time should be negotiated and made available for this.

Alec nodded, and instantly felt for her. And he felt a reaction towards her boss as well, he couldn't help the words 'heartless bastard' that came into his mind. He noted the strength of his reaction. Seemed a bit strong. Mhmm, he thought, perhaps he was straying towards sympathy for his client, taking sides. He needed to be careful. That wasn't his role. Was he feeling too much for his client? Was he making some assumptions here about racism as well? Did he really have grounds to feel that this was racist? He didn't know anything about Merle's boss. He made a mental note to think about this at the end of the session. He needed to offer support to her to be as she wanted to be and not let his feelings towards her boss affect that. And he needed to know why he had such strong feelings too.

'But I do want to come.'

'Yes.' He smiled. 'What do you need to do?'

'I'm going to have to tell him. I mean, I'll say about the bereavement, how it's affected me, perhaps, but I don't really want to say much more.'

'Mhmm, you must say whatever you feel you need or want to say.'

'I'll talk to him and if there are any problems can I give you a ring, otherwise I'll see you next week.'

'Sure. If the answer machine is on, leave a message and if you need me to call you back, give me a time. I'll be discreet if someone else answers.'

'I think I'll leave you my personal mobile number, if that's OK.'

'Sure. Whatever you feel comfortable with.'

Merle gave Alec her number.

'OK. Got that.'

'Thanks.'

'So I hope to see you next week, unless I get a call.'

'Sure. I'm sure it will be OK.' Merle felt her anxiety rising at the thought of it. She got up and took her coat from the hook. 'Thanks.'

'See you next week.'

Merle left feeling lighter in some way. She felt that she had let go of something, even though nothing had been resolved. But having told someone about her manager, somehow that seemed important. She hadn't planned to say anything about it, but she was glad that she had. At the same time, she was aware of wondering whether that disclosure might be passed on, though she also felt sure that it wouldn't. But it was a bit of a nagging worry that she had to consciously push aside. Alec had explained about confidentiality on the phone, and she did feel fairly at ease with him.

She would speak to her boss tomorrow; she knew that she couldn't put it off. At least the building where the staff counselling was sited was close to the unit she worked from, so she could come over fairly easily.

Alec, meanwhile, had begun writing his notes for the session and reflecting on his own reactions to Merle and what she had told him. He also jotted down issues he felt he could usefully take to supervision. It wasn't the first client he had worked with on issues of oppression. At the moment he wasn't sure whether it was racist oppression, or simply oppression, but from what Merle was saying she was the only black nurse in the team and others were confirming to her that she was being given a hard time. He didn't know the track record of her manager. He might be that way towards people for reasons other than colour. Merle had made no comment about there being any definite racist remarks directed towards or about her. Maybe he was that way to new people? Maybe. Or would just single out people irrespective of their skin colour or ethnic background. Maybe again. Mhmm, he didn't know, but he was there to hear Merle's experience.

Clearly, Merle needed to talk, and she hadn't got her aunt now. And he was white, that was the reality and there wasn't any option around that. Yes, in his experience where there was oppression of a black, minority ethnic member of staff by a white person, there was often a racist component so . . . He'd discuss his reaction in supervision. Whether it was oppression or racist oppression, it was unacceptable and Merle had every reason to feel how she was, and every right to address it. It saddened him to think that this continued, but he was also a realist and knew that so much of British society was still riddled with racist attitudes, however much people denied it. And he didn't want to be part of a racist culture.

Points for discussion

- Evaluate Alec's application of the person-centred approach in this session. In particular, how would you describe the quality of his empathy?
- What were the key moments, and how had Alec contributed to them?
- How would you explain confidentiality to a client in this counselling setting?
- What do you need to take special account of in terms of expectations that you, or the client, might have regarding counselling and being counselled by someone from a different ethnic background?
- If you were Alec, what might you consider taking to supervision from this session?
- What are your thoughts, feelings, reactions to racist oppression within the NHS and society generally?
- Write notes for this session.

CHAPTER 2

Counselling session 2: a late cancellation

'Hello, this is a message for Alec from Merle.' The voice sounded anxious and a
little rushed. 'I'm not going to make, it, I'm really, really sorry. We have had
an emergency referral and, well, my manager wants me to go and do a home
visit on this client.' A pause. 'I'm really sorry. Can you call me on my mobile,
you have the number, but in case you haven't here it is again.' The number
followed. 'Can I come next week, I really do need to.' Another pause. 'Sorry,
again.' The sound of the phone hanging up.

Alec stood by the answer phone, pondering the message that had been left whilst
he had been with another client. He felt himself immediately wondering
whether Merle had been singled out because she was planning to come to counselling, or was he becoming a bit paranoid about managers? He didn't know,
but he could hear the anxiety in Merle's voice, and she clearly sounded fed up
about what had happened. He decided to call her back straight away so she
could be immediately reassured that she had another appointment. He got the
answer message on her mobile phone. He guessed she must have it turned off
because of the emergency visit. He couldn't rearrange the time, he was fully
booked through the rest of the day. He left a message.

'Hello, Merle. Alec here from the counselling service. Thanks for your call. Sorry
you are not able to make it but, yes, I can offer you an appointment for the same
time, same day, next week. I hope that will be OK, and that you will be able to
make it. Again, call me if there are any problems.' He hoped that it would sound
OK. Sometimes he felt a bit on the spot with having to record a message. However
much he thought through what he was going to say, there was always something that came to mind and seemed to disrupt the flow of what he was saying.

Alec sat down and thought about it. He needed to put his assumptions aside.
He couldn't risk being in any way partial. Much as there were times when he
had felt like he wanted to tell a client exactly what to do, he knew that it was
usually what he would have wanted to do, and often might not match what the
client wanted or needed to do. And besides, he wanted clients to find their own
voice if that was the issue, and not simply take his voice into a situation.
He hoped that the emergency was genuine and that Merle's manager had no
other choice. He hoped, but he wasn't convinced.

It was after that telephone message that Alec got the call from Merle's boss. 'I gather one of my staff is coming to counselling.' He gave her name. 'So, what's the problem? I can't really afford her the time, so I need to know if it is really important. Something about a bereavement but I thought she'd got over that.'

Alec gritted his teeth as he felt himself react. But he knew that he had to remain calm and focused. He had to ensure confidentiality. He had no agreement with Merle to disclose whether she was attending. He should have done, but he so rarely had managers calling him he had got out of the habit. 'I'm not in a position to confirm or deny whether a member of staff is attending for counselling. Sorry, but we have to protect confidentiality. And if we were seeing someone, we could only confirm this with permission from the staff member.'

The Department of Health (2000, pp. 11–12) publication, *The Provision of Counselling Services for Staff in the NHS* indicates that: 'Confidentiality is crucial to the working relationship. Staff providing counselling will find it beneficial to their work to develop a policy with their colleagues in the personnel/human resources department which is available widely throughout the organisation. Local policies should include explicit references to the guidance relating to confidentiality set out in the 'Code of Ethics and Practice for Counsellors' produced by the British Association for Counselling, guidance produced by the GMC and UKCC and also be consistent with the guidance published by the Department of Health. Counsellors will find it useful to include the following principles in their policy statement so that staff and colleagues are aware of the constraints placed upon the service. These principles apply in all circumstances:

- clients (staff) have a right to expect that counsellors will not disclose any personal information which they learn during the course of their professional duties, unless given permission to do so by the client
- those responsible for confidential information must ensure that the information is effectively protected against improper disclosure when it is disposed of, stored, transmitted or received
- when clients give written consent to the disclosure of information about them, the counsellor must make sure they understand what will be disclosed, the reasons for disclosure and the likely consequences, if any
- counsellors must respect clients' requests that information should not be disclosed to third parties, save in exceptional circumstances (for example where the health and safety of others would be at serious risk). This should be made clear to those who use the service via information leaflets and at the initial meeting
- if confidential information is disclosed, counsellors should release only as much as is necessary for the purpose. Disclosure may be necessary in the public interest where a failure to disclose information may expose the person themselves, a patient, or others, to risk of death or serious harm. Counsellors should make sure that those to whom information

> is disclosed understand that it is given to them in confidence which they must respect
> - if counsellors decide to disclose confidential information they must be prepared to explain and justify their decision.'

'Well I know she's coming, she's told me. God, you counsellors can be so precious. Had one in our team, wouldn't disclose much about the work she was doing.'

'Well, we have a professional boundary to maintain. Usually something appropriate can be negotiated, but clients in counselling have a right to confidentiality.' Alec wasn't, however, going to get into a discussion on the extent of that confidentiality. Equally, he wanted to try and use this contact as an opportunity. 'I can send you some information about the counselling service so you have an idea as to how we work and what we offer.'

'I have it somewhere in my filing cabinet so don't bother.'

'OK.'

'I'll talk to her myself. Can't have staff going off like this and not knowing where they are going. Damned nonsense.'

'I am sorry you feel that way, I am sure it was not intended to cause problems. In my experience staff members do not always want it known that they are attending counselling.'

'Hmm, well, I'll talk to her and call you another time.'

'Like I say, even with a staff member's permission, we would normally only disclose that attendance is taking place.'

Merle's manager muttered a response and hung up.

> Should Alec leave another message for Merle, let her know that her manager has called so that she is aware should her manager speak to her again?

Counselling session 3: motives, demands and exhaustion

There had been no call from Merle and it was now ten minutes before her appointment. Alec was glad and was sitting quietly clearing his thoughts and feelings as was his habit; even after some years of working in a time limited way, he still wondered whether there should be more flexibility. He had worked in other settings where there was a more open-ended arrangement, though he also knew that many people actually chose six sessions and sometimes fewer, finding that they had got what they needed and that they didn't actually want longer term therapy.

The arrangement where he worked was that the eight-session limit would include cancellations, except when there were circumstances quite beyond the client's control, but even then it was hoped that they would let the service know in advance so the slot could be reallocated. Not being allowed to attend because of an emergency in the unit seemed to meet those criteria, and Merle had phoned. Sometimes it felt a little inflexible. But the concern expressed was that the counselling service was a limited resource and that it had to be available to those who wanted, and who needed, it for issues affecting their work performance, or for issues that arose out of work experience. They didn't want the counselling to extend into other areas of a person's life, which Alec accepted could happen once someone began talking.

Alec had always been somewhat sceptical of assessments to decide the number of sessions that a person needed. He didn't naturally work that way. He preferred from a philosophical point of view to allow the client to decide what they felt they needed, and to review and re-negotiate as time went on. But the 'real world', as it had been stated to him on more than one occasion, meant that counselling was limited and had to be targeted.

Anyway, he thought to himself, so often clients start talking about one issue – the 'problem' that has brought them into counselling. It is only later that they then begin to realise that it is linked to other experiences, and the impact they have had on them. They then realise this needs to be addressed if the changes they are wanting or trying to make are to be sustainable. It was something he felt quite passionate about, that sustainable change often (though he accepted not always) could require time. It wasn't that he thought everyone should have lots of time for counselling, that would be unworkable. However, there was something about choice, about employees being treated as responsible adults and of equal status in working out what their needs were.

He tightened his lips as he realised time had passed, and he was supposed to be clearing his mind, not cluttering it up with his own ideas. He took a deep breath and closed his eyes, imagining himself like a mirror, seeing his cloudy emotions thinning and dissolving, and letting his body relax. He liked to go through this little ritual before seeing clients. He felt it helped, and sometimes it would help him identify something that would not clear, some left-over issue that he needed to take to supervision, or perhaps to therapy. But at least it helped him to be aware of it. He recognised the need for ensuring that anything within his sphere of experience was accurately present in his awareness. At least, that was what he aimed for. He knew that in reality this did not always happen, but he did the best that he could.

He opened his eyes, it was time, he got up and went out of the counselling room and down the corridor to the waiting area. Merle was sitting there, looking at her diary. Yes, he thought, how difficult it is to actually switch work off, always something to attend to, something to have to think about, even when you are trying to create space for yourself.

'Hello Merle. You look engrossed!' He smiled.

Merle looked up. 'Oh, hi, yes, just trying to work out when I can make some time to fill in some statistics on my clients. It never ends, does it?'

'Seems not.' Alec paused momentarily. 'Ready to come on through?'

'Sure.' Merle put her diary in her bag and got up, and followed Alec on the short walk down the corridor.

It may not seem like a big issue, but it is worth considering who leads in a situation like this. The client now knows the way. Is it courteous to let them lead? Or should the counsellor lead the way? It is not a matter of there being a 'right' and 'wrong', but that a choice will be made and the counsellor can usefully reflect on their part in that choice. Even at this point, does the person-centred counsellor need to be non-directive? And, if so, how? By asking the client whether they wish to lead? It may seem a small point, but it can bring up issues and as the clarity of self-awareness within the counsellor is important, such a reflection can contribute to raising that self-awareness. If, as some counsellors will experience, there is a long corridor and perhaps a flight of stairs, there are times when it might feel a bit like 'follow-my-leader', and if so, what is that doing to the power relationship between client and counsellor? Also, how much conversation will be appropriate? Issues to reflect on.

'Sorry again about last week.'

'Yes, that's OK. You sounded quite stressed by it on the phone.'

'I was. I really can't believe it happened. And it actually couldn't be helped. There was an emergency assessment needed and I was the only person available. If I'd taken annual leave I'd have been able to get here.'

'So it was one of those unfortunate situations?'

'Yes, a client of mine went psychotic and I had to go out with the psychiatrist. My first reaction was that my boss was playing games, you know, messing me about, but he wasn't. And he agreed to my coming today without it being a problem. It felt a bit out of character, so I'm wondering whether he's worried about what I might be talking about.'

'You think he's feeling under pressure because you're coming to counselling?'

'Something like that. I don't know, or maybe I'm imagining it. Somehow, I can't imagine him being worried, can't imagine him thinking that anyone was having a problem with him, he always gives the impression of knowing he's always right. But, well, if he's worried then good, so long as it doesn't come back at me.'

'You like the idea that he's worried, but, yeah, don't want to suffer from a reaction.'

'No. And I'd really been looking forward to coming last week, to getting away, having some time for me, and in work time as well. That felt good. I need a bit of space. It just seems never ending at the moment. And then there's this Agenda for Change as well, I still don't really understand much about it, but it seems like we're all going to get new job descriptions or something, and salary scales. It's worrying. I can't afford a drop in salary, but no one seems really too sure about it. And Andrew, that's my manager, well, he isn't saying much right now. When anyone mentions it he just brushes it aside, doesn't seem to want to talk about it, just says it's OK, more work for him of course, but he doesn't really say much.'

Alec nodded. He was aware that Agenda for Change was concerning a lot of people, a lot of myths being spread and he knew that he himself didn't feel totally confident what the outcome would be. He knew that some lower paid staff were really worried, and genuinely so, and that there were still discussions with the unions about it. 'So it's been another hectic week and you've got Agenda for Change on your mind as well, and all the uncertainty that it brings.'

Merle nodded. 'Change. Everything just keeps changing these days in the NHS. You can never just stop and take breath, you know? One thing after another.'

'Feels like you can't stop, change all around you in the NHS.'

'Everywhere. And in mental health we are seeing new services, which is great, but they aren't really addressing the problems I'm seeing, you know?'

'So whilst new services are great there's a sense that they aren't helping you much?'

'Well, I mean, the latest is Early Intervention in Psychosis, geared up for 14 year olds upwards; young people and young adults. Identify and treat early, and that's great. Don't get me wrong, we need it, and we need it badly, and we need them to focus on people using substances as well because there's so much drug-induced psychosis, but we get people that simply just keep coming back. Anyone with a problem that can somehow be equated with mental health comes to us, and we've got huge caseloads.' Merle paused, thinking of some of the patients referred to her, more and more who seemed to have become institutionalised into community care, who, the moment they seemed stable and could be discharged, do something – often an act of self-harm or an overdose, and back into hospital and back out to the community team again. She had a few like that and they just could not be moved on.

'So, the early intervention work is good, demand and need for it, but adult services are overburdened with unnecessary referrals.'

'Well, not sure about unnecessary, but people we can't really treat. We get people with border-line personality disorder, and personality disorder that we can't help. We really can't. The psychiatrist prescribes medication to try and keep them stable, but many won't conform to treatment, it's really difficult.'

Alec felt himself react as he hated those terms – personality disorder and border-line personality disorder. It could seem so judgemental. These were terms that often referred to damaged and traumatised people, in his view, whose personalities were disordered for reasons of difficult experiences in their lives. Not always, he accepted that, but he was of the opinion, based on his own work experience, that these kinds of labels could trigger stereotypical reactions, and one that he had come across was the notion that they were untreatable. Maybe the treatment wasn't always appropriate, maybe the setting wasn't right, maybe there wasn't enough time offered, maybe other areas of needed support weren't available. He felt strongly there needed to be more research.

A counsellor may feel strong reactions to something that is said, but unless those reactions seem relevant to the therapeutic process they should be put aside. A counsellor may have strong views, but they are his, and if they affect his ability to give quality attention to his client, then he must take them to supervision. There are other environments for him to pursue and develop his ideas in.

Alec pulled his focus back to Merle. 'So you really struggle with these clients?'

'They need therapy, some of them, or a psychologist, and they need time, you know? We don't have it. The psychology waiting list is enormous, and often they say they're untreatable. It frustrates me. These are people. Yes, I know they can cause chaos sometimes, and some don't conform to treatment, but I have heard stories of abuse and neglect and I'm not surprised it messes people up, really messes them up. We do what we can, but it isn't enough, it just isn't enough.' Merle could feel the frustration rising as she spoke, her voice becoming stronger.

Alec also noticed this and responded to her. 'This really does affect you, I can hear frustration and passion in your voice as well.'

'I want to help these people, that's why I do the job I do, but the system stops us. Too many clients with unrealistic expectations, too many people institutionalised and relying on mental health services. What happened to personal responsibility? Some days all I seem to hear is people expecting me to make them better, and I can't. We do the best we can, and yes, we do help people, but many we really struggle with, you know?'

Alec nodded. 'So many people making demands that you simply cannot satisfy.'

'Don't get me wrong, I like the clients, I do, you know? I'm involved with a service user group and, yeah, that can be challenging, but it's good to sit down with people and hear their suggestions, hear about their difficulties, and it's a group mainly of people who are fairly stable and they feel good about having a voice.'

'So the service user group is a rewarding part of the job for you?'

'It is. Oh, I don't know. It gets to me sometimes and I have to unload. And, well, I wasn't going to say any of that, but now I have.'

'Seems like something you needed to say.'

'It is, but it's not why I'm here.'

Alec noticed a temptation to ask if these work issues were also topics Merle talked to her aunt about, but that would be to direct Merle's focus on to her aunt, and that wasn't his role. He would leave her to find the focus she wanted now that she seemed to be drawing her thoughts and feelings about work to an end.

'Mhmm, you want to focus on something else?'

'Time here is precious. But it is good to sound off, have a bit of a rant, you know? I have group supervision and sometimes it happens there, we have an outside facilitator and that is great. Not all teams have that, but we do and it gives us a chance to talk about not just clients but organisational stuff as well. The team manager doesn't come to it, which is really good.'

Alec caught a look in Merle's eyes that seemed to reflect a certain wickedness. He could only imagine what may get said.

'So you talk about clients, the organisation and the team manager.'

'Yeah, he's such a miserable bastard.'

Alec wondered what mechanisms there were for the topics of the supervision group to be fed back into the line-management process. But he wasn't going to direct the focus to that. He knew from his own experience that often there would be some kind of mechanism so that issues that needed to be addressed could be picked up by someone more senior.

'Mhmm, miserable bastard.'

'I'm back talking about work again, and I don't want to do that, but it just seems so much with me at the moment.'

'Mhmm, work is really present.'

> The counsellor has offered a series of short and focused empathic responses. It has enabled the client to flow with what is in her thoughts, and she has stayed with aspects of her work with clients and her supervision group, even though she has questioned if she wants to use the time to talk about that. She is saying what she needs to say, and experiencing a certain sense of feeling she should talk about something else. The overwhelming presence of work is therefore emerging.

'I guess it's because I'm off to see a client after this, and then we have a clinical meeting, there's so few gaps in the diary, so little time to stop and think, you know? We're supposed to have time for reading and professional development, and it gets swallowed up time and time again.'

Alec noticed how quickly Merle was speaking. 'I'm just aware how quickly you are talking, it's like there's no time to slow down.'

'Sorry.'

'No, I didn't mean it like a criticism, but an observation of how it is, you know?' Alec smiled inwardly, he realised he'd picked up on Merle's habit of saying 'you know'.

> Alec's intervention has momentarily interrupted the flow, but he has been able to explain his meaning. It emerges that what he said was right, but the client wasn't, in that moment, in a place in herself to acknowledge it, his comment put her – or should we say she reacted to his comment – by feeling she had maybe done something wrong for which she had to apologise. In a sense it indicates her sensitivity to another person's perception of her. It may well be indicative of her external locus of evaluation having some dominance.

'Yeah, but it's like that. I get so keyed up. Look at me, I'm so tense. Jesus.' Merle moved her shoulders, feeling the tension in them as she tried to relax for a moment.

'Really gets into your body.'

Merle shook her head, 'some evenings I go home and I don't think I really do wind down. And if mum's having a bad one, well, actually I usually go out, try and meet up with friends. A few drinks help.'

Alec nodded. 'Helps you relax, yeah?'

'Yeah, and I keep tabs on it. But yeah, it does help.'

'It's important to have ways of relaxing.'

'Yeah, and that's why I miss auntie Jessie. She slowed everything down, that was her way. She was just slow, know what I mean?'

'Her manner, you mean?'

'Her everything. She'd look at me and say, "why you running about like a headless chicken? You just slow down. You don't need to rush. I never rushed, just take life slowly, carefully. Crazy people rush around, you don't need to." Yeah, she slowed me down.' Merle had a head full of memories, of sitting with her aunt, sometimes in her front room, other times in the kitchen. She'd sit there for hours sometimes, just the two of them. Her brother'd be there when they were younger some of the time. Good times to share. She felt the lump in her throat as she thought of her aunt's face, her smile, her eyes that seemed to sparkle with mischief. She'd tell her stories about her past and make her laugh. She missed that, she missed it all. Now it felt like she was on her own. On her own . . . The sadness was back with her again.

'Quite a woman, your aunt . . .' Alec spoke slowly and deliberately having sensed the change of mood.

'She used to tell me that I was doing a good job, that I was a natural for caring about people.' Merle smiled although her eyes were watery.

'Caring about people's important to you?'

Merle nodded. 'Yeah, deep down, I do what I do because I care about people, you know, I like to help people and, well, nursing just seemed right for me. Couldn't just work in an office, lot of friends from school became hairdressers or typists, that kind of thing. But I didn't just want to be with people, I always felt I wanted to care, wanted to look after people. So I started off in general nursing. I really liked that but realised I was becoming more and more interested in the psychology of illness, that kind of thing. I suppose it came out of talking to people. I used to get into trouble, spending too much time talking to patients, but I was interested in them. I wanted to hear about their lives and, well, people say I'm a good listener. So, yeah, I trained in psychiatric nursing and I really do like it, it's just that, well, things aren't so good at the moment.'

'Yes. Wanting to care.'

'More than that. Wanting to make a difference. I want to help people claim a better life for themselves, and some do, and it's so great to see. Not everyone does, as I said we see so many people who just seem stuck, they can't seem to move on, and we can't seem to help them, for whatever the reason. But it's great when you help someone get some control back in their lives, help them make sense of their illness, help them get themselves into something more fulfilling, you know? Yeah, it's about making a difference for people.'

'Mhmm, making a difference.'

Merle thought for a moment, 'and it gets harder because it feels like more and more people are stuck, and if you don't get a sense of making that difference, well, it makes it harder, you know?'

'Harder to . . . ?'

'. . . to keep going, I guess, keep motivated. But that's on a bad day. On a good day, well, it's OK.'

'Mhmm, so it's OK on a good day, you feel you're making a difference, you feel positive, but on a bad day . . .'

'On a bad day it's like too much, just too much.'

Merle lapsed into silence. She felt a little bit talked out. When she spoke again it was in a much quieter voice. 'Yeah, I care about my patients. I just want to make a difference.' And she thought of how difficult some of her patients were, and how with some of them it really felt like damage limitation – contain and control. There were some damaged people out there, she thought to herself, many had been abused in one way or another in their lives – either as a result of mental illness, but often it seemed to be part of the cause. She took a deep breath and sighed.

'You care about the people you want to make a difference with.'

'Yeah. And sometimes I wonder why. Sometimes I'm in a place where I really do question if it's really worth it, you know?'

'Really worth . . . ?'

'Worth the effort, worth the stress, worth the exhaustion. There are a lot of people like me working in the NHS, dedicated and utterly exhausted.'

Alec knew she was right. He nodded. 'I know.' He paused and then continued, realising he had spoken for himself and not empathised with Merle. 'But it leaves you wondering if it is worth it.'

'I know it is, I don't think I could do anything else, but maybe somewhere without the pressure and the demands. I do feel like I'm being exploited sometimes, it's like we're under-resourced but still expected to do what we have always done, only with more patients and more complexity.' Merle shook her head. 'I really do feel like we are taken advantage of.' She lapsed into silence.

Alec nodded again, he knew that one too. It was a problem that he heard and witnessed many times, people feeling taken advantage of, a kind of emotional blackmail – no, maybe that was too strong – but certainly a sense that people's caring was not just being used, or over-used, but actually abused. Staff being expected to do that little bit more to make it easier for patients, at whatever cost to them. Too many staff ended up as patients – not necessarily in mental health services, but generally, developing illnesses themselves, stress-related symptoms, people burning out, reaching that point where they feel they have given all they can, that there is nothing left, reaching a point at which they quite literally fold under the pressure, or perhaps *crumple* would be a better word, yes, crumple under the strain of it all. And more and more NHS workplace counsellors being brought in to try and prop people up, keep them going a little longer. Or was he being cynical? Well, he probably was, but he also felt there was a truth in it as well.

It is recognised that the NHS is an organisation that is stressful to work for. Alec witnesses this daily and it has become something that is very present for him in his thoughts and his feelings. When Merle describes this he slips into his own inner world. Of course, as a result, he will have disconnected from his client. This highlights the issue for a counsellor of how to cope with hearing something similar many times over, and in very emotional and personal ways that are bound to have had an effect. It is as though a group of thoughts and feelings develop within the counsellor's awareness which is then accessed when a client describes an experience that in some sense resonates to what is already present for the counsellor.

In NHS settings where there can be similarities of issues brought to counselling this needs to be monitored carefully and where disconnection from the client occurs to a significant degree, this needs exploring in supervision.

Merle's voice brought Alec away from his thoughts.

'Sometimes I wonder if I'd be better off getting out and working for a nursing agency – better money, less hassle, less commitment. But then, I don't know, somehow it doesn't seem right. I like to feel part of a team, not someone who comes and goes. I like to work over time with clients and that can't be guaranteed with an agency.'

'Mhmm, more money, less hassle but lose out on that longer term contact with clients.'

Merle listened to Alec's response, and somehow it left her feeling a little more in favour of getting out, particularly the hassle factor, but then she knew there could be hassle anywhere. Still, at least with agency work it's easier to move on. But she liked her work colleagues. They really did try and work as a team, not because of the manager, but really for their own survival. But a couple of the nurses had left in recent months and that had been unsettling, and she had felt it particularly when Andrea had left. They'd joined at about the same time, in fact they'd trained around the same time though in different places. She remembered thinking when Andrea announced she was leaving, 'damn, she's found a way out'. It had really left her wondering what she was doing. She'd talked to her aunt about it, and whilst she had been sympathetic she had encouraged her to stay. She didn't really know why, other than that was her aunt's way. 'Don't make changes until you have to, until you're really sure. Better the devil you know ...' she'd say. Well Merle knew the devil alright, and at times it got her down, at times she wanted to walk away from it, and at other times, on good days, it felt like no devil at all.

'I need a break, that's for sure. Maybe I need to take a week off soon. I haven't any leave planned, maybe I need to take time out and go away somewhere.' She thought about who she might go with, find some cheap package holiday and some sunshine.

'Mhmm, leaves you feeling you want to take some holiday, get away.' Alec smiled inwardly, wondering if Merle's sensed need to get away would, in time, develop into a clearer need to leave her current job. But that was speculation. He'd seen it happen. People under stress deciding that they didn't need to put up with it any more. He didn't sense Merle was in that place.

'I know it won't change anything, but it would give me something to look forward to in a few weeks, and, who knows, maybe I'd feel better afterwards. And a few more counselling sessions as well, maybe . . .' She smiled at Alec.

> The client, having been allowed to explore freely what she is thinking and feeling, has connected with a sensed need for a break. It is not something that has been suggested to her, or that she has been directed towards, it has naturally emerged in response to her experience of herself and of her options. It is therefore likely to be highly timely and trustworthy as a course of action for the client to take. She feels she has had enough, the idea of something new appeals, but that's a big step. The idea of a break, of time away, simply makes sense and it would be reasonable to suggest that it probably, in the moment of thinking about it, is making Merle feel good. That is a powerful motivation for her to act on her idea.

Alec smiled back. The clock had caught his eye a moment or two before. 'Time's nearly up. You've said a lot today, not so much upset as last week, but things you feel passionate about. I hope it has been helpful.'

Merle nodded. 'I didn't think I'd talk this way, but it has been good to get it off my chest. When I think of the kind of jobs that other people do, I really wonder why I put myself through it. But then I think of patients that have got things together, who have maybe resolved their depression, or made changes in their lives and reduced their levels of anxiety; or people that have resolved their need to self-harm and have made a bit of a fresh start, then I know why. But I can't keep on, not without getting something back.'

'And sometimes the successes aren't quite enough.'

Merle nodded again. Yes, she thought, that was the truth of it. Sometimes, however much she cared, however much she wanted to make a difference, there just weren't enough successes to counter-balance the stresses, the demands and the exhaustion, the feeling of giving so much and there still being more demanded when it seemed she had nothing left. Those were the days when she went home feeling utterly despairing of it all. Everything was an effort. She so wanted to be able to work without those days. The difficulty was that they seemed to be all too frequent.

'Well, I'll survive I'm sure. I never did stop talking about work, did I?'

'Not really.'

'It's been good. Good to get it out.'

'Mhmm.'

'So, same time next week?'

'Sure, no problem.'

Merle got up and left. She didn't feel quite the same as the previous week. She didn't feel that lightness, she actually felt more weighed down. She had to rush to her appointment. She made a mental note to try and spend time that evening thinking about the counselling session. She didn't want to lose it in the general rush of demand on her.

Alec felt exhausted after the session. So much, he thought to himself, so much. And he heard it again and again from mental health workers, struggling with heavy caseloads, complex clients, difficulties coping with clients for whom it seemed there were no resources – or services – that could meet their needs. And he knew as well that however exhausted he felt, Merle would be feeling it more acutely still. Maybe she had managed to unload some of it in the session. She had certainly brought it into the room, even though much of the time she had talked quite fast. But there had been a lot of silences, a lot of times when she had clearly been with her own thoughts, brought to places in herself through the dialogue and the themes that emerged.

He didn't feel that he had said a great deal. He hoped that Merle had said what she needed to say, that he hadn't unwittingly directed her into areas that were of particular interest to him. He didn't think that he had, but he knew how easy it was to have blind spots. He opened his file, wrote in the date and began to write his notes for the session, again jotting down issues that he felt he wanted to take to supervision.

Points for discussion

- What strikes you from the session and how are you left feeling?
- Do you feel that Alec communicated empathy effectively? How did he convey warm acceptance? Find examples.
- What would you be taking to supervision if you were Alec?
- If you were giving Merle advice, what would it be? How would you ensure you do not do this as a counsellor?
- Write notes for this session.

CHAPTER 3

Counselling session 4: the client is seeking her own voice

Merle was sitting in the waiting room – she had arrived a few minutes early, glad to make use of the opportunity to get away. It had been a hectic morning once again and she was feeling fed up. She always seemed to get allocated the more complex cases, at least that was how it felt, although she wasn't alone in that view. She had needed to discuss two of her patients with the psychiatrist and she had commented on how many complex cases she seemed to have. It had rekindled Merle's feelings of being picked on. Another thing that had come up during the week was the issue of training. The service had a very limited training budget and whilst others had been to external conferences, Merle hadn't, although she had expressed interest. It wasn't something new to her. She had experienced the same kind of what felt to her like discrimination in her previous job – it had been part of her reason for leaving. Once again, she had been passed over. She'd wanted to complain more vociferously, but she could hear her aunt's voice in her head, 'keep you head down, girl, get on with your work, it'll all work out'. Strangely enough her reaction had not simply been to accept what her aunt had said, rather she felt quite angry towards her. That was a new experience. She was pondering on it once again when she heard Alec call her name.

Alec stood aside and let Merle lead the way to the counselling room. Having sat down he asked her how she wanted to use the time that day. She still had her aunt's voice in her head, and a feeling of anger, a sense of wanting more but at the same time shrinking back from making a noise about it.

'I just don't seem to get what my colleagues do, I get passed over on things.'

Alec maintained his focus on Merle, 'so things get offered to others but not to you, that how it is?' He sensed what was being said was important and he wanted to be sure that both Merle and he fully appreciated the nature of the problem.

> An example of empathy used to clarify what is being communicated by the client. Different words are used and there is a tentative, questioning tone, a

> checking out quality. This enables the client to feel heard and, at the same, leaves an opportunity for taking time to really be clear as to what is being experienced.

'Yeah, like there's a conference coming up and it would be good for me to go on it, you know, it's about the new mental health act and what it means, and it's something I could usefully bring back to the team. But no, someone else is picked. OK, so he's more senior in the team, but he often goes to conferences, but it should be spread around. I'm experienced too, maybe not so long in the team as others, but I've got a number of years experience of working in mental health but somehow that seems forgotten.'

'So your experience is overlooked or forgotten.'

'It's like I'm not valued for what I have to offer.'

'Mhmm, you have a lot to offer but there's no sense that it is valued.'

Merle took a deep breath. 'And I used to talk about this with my aunt, and she'd tell me not to worry, so long as I was doing a good job, that was all that mattered. Told me that it was God's will and I should do my job as well as I could.' She shook her head. 'I now really am beginning to wonder about that.'

'Wonder about ...?'

'God's will. I don't know. It doesn't seem right and, well ... Oh, I don't know.'

'It sounds troubling, hard to make sense of.' Alec sought to empathise with the struggle in Merle's thoughts, leaving it open for her to develop them as she felt she needed.

'I mean, I've as much right to represent the service at a conference, and I really feel ...' She couldn't find the right words. She was experiencing a whole mixture of feelings as she sat, shaking her head with Alec looking on.

'You really feel ...' Alec left his response unfinished, empathising with what had been said and offering the opportunity for Merle to try and express what she was feeling.

'... like I really do want to make a noise, you know. I'm fed up being, I don't know, given the rubbish jobs.'

'Mhmm, you want to make a noise. You're fed up with being given the rubbish jobs, yeah?'

'Yes, I am. And I want things to be different. I want a bit of respect, that's what it is.' She felt strong and determined – it felt good.

'Mhmm, respect for ...?' Again Alec left his response open to allow Merle to clarify.

'Respect for me as a nurse, but more than that, respect for me as a person, you know, respect for my colour, respect for my commitment, my professionalism, for how much I give to my job, my patients, the team.' She was looking up at Alec now, and shaking her head. 'And I know it may sound a bit of a cliché, respect, but it really does sum it up. I really do feel like I'm seen by some people as "the little black nurse", and I'm fed up with it.'

Alec heard what Merle was saying and briefly wondered what his view was. Did he fall into the same category of person? How did he view Merle? Something to ponder on ... The way Merle spoke really communicated to him a sense of the put down, of the oppressive nature of that kind of attitude. The word was strong in his mind and yet he felt strongly that it was his word, and that maybe he needed to help Merle find her own language for what she was experiencing. Or maybe she already had?

The counsellor could respond here by saying something like, 'it gives me a sense of how oppressive it must feel for you', but is this therapeutically helpful? Would it not be more valuable for the client to acknowledge it in those terms? Or maybe she doesn't need to, she knows what it feels like, she's been there for much of her working life. She doesn't need some white man to talk about oppression, it's part of her experience. Only now she is perhaps beginning to relate differently to it, to discover or rather engage more fully with how she feels about it, questioning her aunt's attitude of accepting it.

Stop for a moment, if you are a white counsellor reading this, and imagine how patronising and pathetic it might sound for you to say, 'sounds like you're feeling oppressed'. Black minority ethnic people live with this on a daily basis in many areas of life. It's a constant, in the background, and in the foreground of their lives as well.

Having said the above, there will also be times when it will be therapeutically valuable for the client to hear the counsellor acknowledge the existence of oppression. But it needs to be voiced sensitively in the cases where the counsellor is ethnically a member of the oppressing group.

Alec decided to stay with a straight empathic reflection of the words Merle had used, seeking to place similar emphasis on the words to the way that Merle had spoken them. 'Yeah, fed up with being seen by some people as "the little black nurse".' He didn't say anything more. He wanted to somehow respect Merle as a person, a woman, yes as a person of colour. But he didn't know quite what else to say. Then it came to him, and it felt right, 'and, you know, as a white man in this culture, I need to learn more about what that means. But I don't want my stuff to take you away from the strength of what you feel, and rightly so.'

Merle looked at Alec, trying to make him out. He'd listened to her these past few weeks, she felt that he was there for her in some way, that he didn't think like she knew some other men and women did. 'It's always there, Alec, it's always there.'

Alec nodded. 'I know.' He really did feel a heavy heart as he responded. Yes, he did know. His counselling training had been with a group of people with a wonderful mix of ethnic background, and he was aware that it had been a really important experience for him to train and work with such a diverse group. He felt so frustrated when he heard about all-white, middle-class training groups that took place in some parts of the country. Groups where he feared the reality of oppression because of race and ethnicity could never be really brought into the training arena. For him it had been a factor throughout his training, and he had so valued how helpful it had been to be getting perspectives from people of different racial backgrounds on how racism and oppression impacted on their experience in the context of the different topics they covered. And he was gay and that had brought him his own experience of oppression. He knew that there were counsellors who were quite out of touch with the reality of race, culture, diversity and ethnicity issues. And he had recognised through his training and therapy that he, too, carried prejudices. He didn't like the idea when he was challenged over it, but came to realise that they were present. But he felt that he had worked them through and yet, even now, he could still catch himself experiencing greater anxiety when walking along a street and encountering a group of black youths in contrast to feelings when seeing a group of white youths.

Merle felt herself thinking, yes, I think you do know, the look in your eyes tells me that you do, and yet I also know that unless you wear my skin colour, you cannot really know. But she didn't feel confident in saying that and she let the thought go.

'And you know, I guess I really want it to stop, but it's so big, it's so everywhere.'

Alec nodded again. He could feel himself shifting into sympathy but pulled himself back into his awareness of what Merle had said, and empathised with her. 'Yes, you want it to stop, to not be there, but it's just everywhere.'

'Do you think it'll ever change, I mean, really change?'

Alec felt himself momentarily wonder whether Merle was asking for an answer, or wanted to be held with the question. His sense was that it was more of a question to him, seeking a response. 'I hope so, I truly hope so.'

'I mean, sometimes I think it just gets worse. With friends, yeah, I don't think it's there, we all get on just fine, you know, and I've got white friends, Asian friends, people with all kinds of mixed ethnic backgrounds. But at work, in an organisation, when you come up against people you don't know personally, really know, that is, then it's there.'

'It's like personal relationships can sort of, I don't know, rise above it – and I'm not sure if those are the right words – but where people don't know you they sometimes can't see beyond skin colour.'

'And your voice, on the phone. I mean, I've still got some accent, you know.'

'So have I!' Alec smiled. 'Sorry, but in a small way I've felt my accent has been a problem, but I'm not going to compare it to your experience.'

'But you're right, people can't see beyond the obvious: looks, voice. And then they don't relate to you, as a person, but to some idea they have in their head.'

'And that's what you have to battle with daily.'

'Truth is, I don't think I have battled, just put up with it, accepted it.' Merle was shaking her head again. 'That was my aunt's attitude, bless her. She was quite old, I guess it was a generational thing. I mean she was 70 when she died. She was the oldest of my mother's siblings; my mother was the youngest, so in a way they were almost a generation apart.'

'Mhmm, so your aunt took the view of accepting it, and you feel you adopted that?'

Merle was nodding. 'I don't want to be critical of her, I loved her, she was so important for me, you know?'

It was Alec's turn to nod. 'I can sense that from the way you speak about her, a lot of love, a lot of respect.'

'And I do miss her, but I also begin to wonder whether she was right. Maybe right for her, maybe, I don't know. But maybe not right for me.'

'Mhmm, maybe her words were right for her generation, or for her in her past in some way, but you now question whether they are right for you, now.'

'I want to agree with her, but I don't think I can, not any more. I really don't.'

'Not prepared to accept the way some people treat you because of your colour any more.' He emphasised the last two words as this seemed to be an area that Merle was emphasising.

Merle took a deep breath. 'So what now? In a job, constant demands, stressful, exhausting, feeling I'm treated differently because of my colour, feeling I'm losing out on opportunities.' She looked down. 'In spite of all I've said, I still find it hard to think of doing anything about it. I guess the truth is I don't know what to do.'

'Mhmm. It's not easy, feeling pulled in two different directions.' Alec empathised with the sense of Merle's dilemma that he felt she was communicating to him.

It could be argued that Alec has not empathised with the really important part of what has been said by Merle – the not knowing what to do. This can be difficult to empathise with when the counsellor also feels a sense of powerlessness. An 'avoidance' can take place, where counsellor and client collude to keep a distance from some painful reality. However, Merle is engaging with her sense of not knowing what to do, she is verbalising it, and Alec has not empathised with it. Sometimes a client will repeat a statement because it is important, and may continue to do so until the counsellor shows that he has heard them; at other times the client may give up and move on to something else, or be unwittingly directed to something else by the counsellor.

The person-centred counsellor will want to stay with the client, with the difficulty and, in this case, with the simple fact of not knowing what to do and the feelings and thoughts that this arouses.

'I guess I am pulled, but in a way I know I have to do something. It's not knowing quite what and wondering if I have the courage to do something about it.'

'The "what do I do?", and if I decide what to do, will I have the courage to follow it through?'

'Sitting here it's kind of easy, in a way, to talk about it. But doing it. What do I do, go up to my manager and tell him he's a racist bastard?' Merle stared ahead of her. 'Part of me wants to do that, but I can already feeling myself shrinking back from it.'

'Yes, you'd really like to tell him how it is, tell him he's a racist bastard, but the thought of doing that ...'

'... I can feel myself wanting to, I don't know, but there's a voice in my head saying, "no, no, you don't want to do that"; but I do, and maybe I have to. Maybe not quite like that, but maybe I do need to say something.'

'So that sounds clear, although it makes you uncomfortable thinking about it, there is a sense that you feel you really do need to say something.'

Merle thought about what Alec was saying. 'If I let it go again, well, it just goes on, doesn't it? And, well, if it gets horrible, I can always get another job.' She hesitated, and as she continued her voice was stronger. 'But I don't want that. Why should I have to change my job? No, I like the people I work with, the clinicians, we work really well together. I need to say something, and I need to think of the best way of saying it.'

'Mhmm, so you want to say something, you plan to say something, it's finding the right words.'

'It won't help if I get angry, and I can't back down either once I've said it.'

'The Trust has a zero tolerance policy on racism, Merle, and they can bring in someone to mediate in these situations.'

'I know, and maybe it will come to that, but I think for now I need to maybe make a list of what has happened to me, what my grievances are, and then, well, then I'll decide once I see it written down.'

'Sounds like a very positive and realistic step to take.' Alec was genuine in his response. It wasn't an easy thing to contemplate. It wasn't always easy for people to confront their manager about their behaviour. He wished that more organisations adopted more of a 360-degree appraisal system, it could provide opportunity for problems or issues to come to light. It wasn't the answer to everything, grievance procedures were in place and well established. The difficulty was always when the person who felt oppressed simply couldn't find the confidence to actually take action. But he sensed that Merle had changed since she had started to come to counselling, that she was now finding her voice, and moving away from accepting her lot, as it were, to accepting her need to challenge it and those who perpetuated the oppression that she was feeling.

In 360-degree appraisal a member of staff seeks feedback from those above and below them in their organisation, as well as from peers and sometimes people from outside agencies with whom they have partnership-working. This is then reviewed by a more senior manager and fed back to the person being appraised.

'Yes, I'll do that. I'll type up a list. Maybe I should have been keeping a record before, but I hadn't thought about it in the way that I am now.'

'Mhmm, so make the list and then think about what to do next.'

'I don't really want to take out a grievance, it seems so heavy somehow, and yet, I mean, I wonder ... , oh I don't know.'

'Mixed feelings?'

'Just uncertainty about what's best, and feeling anxious about doing it.'

'Yes, hard to get away from those feelings.'

'I guess I could easily begin to doubt myself. That's where I think I need the list. I need to have a record of the things that make me feel like I'm being singled out.'

Alec nodded. 'You have a base then, a kind of foundation.'

'I need that.' Merle took a deep breath before continuing. 'I never expected to be contemplating this when I first came here. I was in a very different place, I really was.'

'I know. You couldn't have considered any of this. But it seems that now you are ready to confront the issue. It seems like you are wanting to find a voice, your voice, in all of this.'

'Yes, and I wonder how that will be because it doesn't feel easy to think about.'

'No. No. Sometimes it is easier to set these kinds of grievance off out of a burst of anger, when you simply have had enough, can't take any more, and want to make a very loud noise about it.'

'And I suppose that's fine, you don't give yourself a chance to think about it.' Merle paused, collecting her thoughts. 'I do want to think about it, but that's the problem, thinking about it makes me aware of how big it all feels, and how small it can make me feel.'

'Yes, but the Trust takes this kind of issue seriously.'

'I hope so, but I do wonder. Not many senior, I mean really senior people, are black. You look in the Trust newsletter and any pictures of really senior people, and they're nearly all white.'

'Yes, doesn't help, does it?'

Somehow both Alec and Merle had lost track of the time, and the session was almost due to end. 'Time's sped past, Merle, so you're going to make a list and then take it from there?'

'I'll see how I get on. Not sure when I'll get a chance to do it, and maybe I'll talk about it next week.'

'Fine, no problem, bring it with you if you want, up to you, see how it goes.'

'Sure that's OK?'

'Yes, it'll be fine.'

Merle got up and left. She felt a little wobbly as she went along the corridor. She felt as though she had just made a big commitment, and already she was wondering whether she could carry it through. But she knew she had to, she couldn't shrink back from it, not now. She'd list her grievances, talk it through with Alec next week, and then . . . Hmm, she thought, and then . . .

Alec sat back in his chair. Yes, Merle was doing what she needed to do, and counselling was helping her to do it. He smiled as he thought about just how revolutionary counselling was, or could be, in the NHS workplace. So often people were referred to counselling so they could get back to work or improve their work performance, but so often he found his clients were actually seeking something else, something deeper, more immediate and personal. All kinds of issues brought people into the counselling room, but the topics that were then discussed could leave people feeling very different about themselves, their work, the NHS. No wonder so many counselling services seemed to be set up to keep the focus specifically on the presenting issue. Yes, he did wonder sometimes about the real motive behind staff counselling. Was it only to patch people up and keep them going? Or was he being somewhat disingenuous in his thinking? Maybe he was. The problem was, as he saw it, in reality you cannot truly separate out a work-related issue from other aspects of a person's life. People are people, made up of complex relationships, with parts of their lives and of themselves overlapping. Change one area and it impacts on other areas. To think you can in some sort of precise way simply address one area of a person's being in isolation was absurd. And yet, people did benefit from staff counselling, and often clients would seek further counselling to look at other areas of themselves and their lives. Ah well, he thought, long live the revolution, particularly the person-centred one with its philosophy of non-directiveness and belief in the power of the individual to find their own solutions rather than be reliant on external experts.

Points for discussion

- How is Alec bringing himself into the therapeutic relationship? Is he being effective in this way?
- How did you respond to the dialogue regarding oppression and racism? What are the issues that a counsellor needs to consider and resolve within themselves in order to be able to work effectively on these issues?
- Where would you have responded differently to Merle in counselling session 4, and what would have informed your different responses?
- Contrast Merle at the end of this session with how she presented in the first session. What has changed and what has enabled that change to take place?
- What might you take to supervision from this session, and why?
- Alec has experienced homophobic reactions to him being a gay man. Contrast this with someone experiencing racist oppression and the effect it might have on their developing self-concept.
- Write notes for this session.

CHAPTER 4

Supervision session 1: colour, racism, oppression and language

Alec had been working with Bernadette, his supervisor, for three years now. He greatly appreciated her down to earth way of being. She also brought a strong Afro-Caribbean quality into her work and this Alec found quite refreshing. He had worked with a number of supervisors and liked to move on every four or five years, sometimes earlier, depending on circumstances. He found it enriching to establish collaborative relationships with different people. It was also extremely helpful because Bernadette had experience of working in the NHS herself, as a counsellor, and had an appreciation of what the NHS could be like, the pressures and the stresses. He knew not everyone felt a background knowledge of a situation to be important, but he certainly found it helpful at times.

He had already given her Merle's history, and the issues that were arising.

'So, you're working with oppression. How does that feel?' Bernadette knew she was provoking Alec, and she wanted him to react. She wanted to be sure that he was owning his own stuff and was therefore clear and present for his client.

'Uncomfortable. Brings up a lot of feelings and thoughts.'

'Such as?'

'About being white, about being seen as one of the oppressors because of my skin colour.'

'Mhmm. Not nice to feel a particular way because of the colour of your skin.'

'No. It's not new, the issue has come up before, as you know.'

'Mhmm, but it's important to explore it, helps to keep us sharp.'

'I know.'

Bernadette sat and waited for Alec to maybe say a little more. She knew he was uncomfortable, and she knew he was the kind of guy who wanted to be honest with himself, and do the best he could with his clients.

'I suppose there are a few issues here for me. One is to do with the risk of siding with the client – partly because of the issue; her manager does sound like, what did Merle, say, a miserable bastard, something like that. I know I had a strong reaction to him quite early on, which left me thinking I was straying towards too much sympathy for Merle. I know I don't like oppression, or racism, but I also know I can't start allowing this to cause me to take sides. At least I noticed it. And, well, he's also phoned me as well, which I think just reinforced my feelings. But I know I have to, well, acknowledge they are there but I can't let them cloud the accuracy of my empathy for my client.' Alec paused for a moment before continuing.

'Anyway, he phoned to try to get information. I felt myself react straight away, but kept my cool. But also partly as a result of maybe over-compensating for feelings I may have as a white man working with a black woman on issues of racism and oppression.'

'Mhmm. Good. Both really important to have in mind.'

'I don't think I'm siding with her, well, I'm feeling on her side, but I don't think I'm leading her. But, I have to self-monitor and be open to that possibility. These are strong issues that touch into, well, for me, my identity and how I want to be in the world, and how I want to be perceived as well. I genuinely think she is finding her own feelings, making her own decisions and, yes, beginning to find her own voice.'

'Mhmm, yes, you think Merle's finding her own way. But you are open to the need to self-monitor around taking sides as an effect of over-compensation.'

'That's how it feels to me. And it's good to be able to acknowledge it. But that's not enough, I know that. I have to keep my empathy accurate, my congruence clear and my positive regard unconditional or in some way influenced or affected – and I was about to say "coloured" and maybe, somehow, that is the right word to use. I know it may sound a bit of a Freudian slip, but I think there's a truth here as well. You know?'

'Do you want to explore that further?' Bernadette felt that this was perhaps in need of further exploration now that it had been raised. She wanted to be sure Alec's client felt she could say what she wanted, be how she needed to be, and feel respected as a woman, a professional, a person of a particular colour and culture.

'It's like, my issues around diversity exist. I have my experiences, my views, how I believe myself to be which is what I hope others experience as well. I don't like racism and I don't like oppression. We're all people and I want to celebrate cultural diversity. I value difference. I don't want to feed into a view that somehow sees it as a threat in some way to my culture. We're a multi-cultural world – fact.'

'Not everyone feels that way.'

'No, mhmm, and I guess I want to . . .' Alec paused. 'Why am I trying so hard?'

'Why do you think?'

'Because I'm not sure that I am going to be perceived as I want to be perceived.'

'Because?'

'Maybe I'm not so accepting of cultural diversity as I think I am or want to be?' He stopped and reflected further on what he had said. Was that right? Well, yes, he had to be honest and say so. 'Yes, I'm afraid that something will get out, make me . . . mhmm. And I know as well that there are times when I am sure I make some comment and it probably will have some racist side to it. It's not meant to be that way, but ... Years of conditioning, I suppose, being brought up in a very white area. I actually think I've adapted well, but, yes, there is that doubt. And that's something I need to explore further, here, in therapy, to think through for myself. And it isn't new, I know that this is how it can be. And I'm grateful in a way that this is drawing my attention to something maybe in me. I can learn from this, weed it out. So long as I make sure it doesn't have a non-therapeutic effect on my client.' Alec paused again. 'Not sure where to go with this now, feels like I have acknowledged something and must give it more thought, and I'm aware of other areas I want to focus on today. I'd like to leave it at that, and come back to it after I've given it more thought myself, and I may take it into therapy if I need to, but I'm not sure about that, I need to process it more myself.'

'OK. I leave that with you, and you know you can bring anything you need to hear on this because it is a supervision issue as well in terms of it being something that could impact on what you're offering clients.'

Alec nodded in response. Yes, he knew that. He needed to take another look at this issue.

Bernadette appreciated Alec's striving to be honest with himself for the benefit of his clients. She knew she could trust him to work on himself. She well appreciated how deep seated and subtle racist attitudes and values could be, and that they weren't all dealt with in training and therapy, that they could bubble out later. What was important was that they could be acknowledged openly and honestly, and explored with a view to being able to resolve them.

'So, going back to my client's relationship with her aunt, I feel I've lost my thread a bit here.'

'From what you said it seems like her aunt had a major role in her life and, from what you were saying earlier, now she's starting to question some of her aunt's wisdom. That's a tough place to be.'

Alec nodded, 'yes, yes, that's right, and I do respect that. The one person who has been such a support and then you begin to find yourself questioning some of the things they have said. I wonder, you know, whether she is going to be able to carry forward her plan to talk to her boss about what has been happening.'

'You think the oppressed part of her that wants a quiet life might take control again?'

'Well, she's at an early stage of questioning, and of allowing another way of being to emerge. The old way is likely to fight back, as it can.'

Bernadette nodded. 'Yes, not easy to think differently and behave differently, and particularly when she will feel a strong allegiance to her aunt. Family is important, you know? And in some cultures more than others.'

'Yet from what I've picked up – and Merle hasn't really talked much about her family, not really. I know she has a brother but they're not close, the father is hardly mentioned, and her mother, well, she seems to have her own problems.'

'And Merle lives with her mother?'

'Yes, but it's not easy. I think Merle goes out with friends, likes a few drinks to relax. I have a feeling she said something about how her mother is – I think it may be depression, certainly mood problems.'

'So her aunt was maybe a bit of a parent as well?'

'Seems like it.'

'And no mention of grandparents?'

'No, but if her mother's sister died recently at 70, well, they're very likely no longer alive.'

'No, no, quite an age gap, but not unusual. Big families, you know.'

'Yes, and it's interesting that Merle has said very little about anything related to her family. I mean, I don't ask, I don't do that kind of assessment. I want her to tell me what she wants me to hear, what she wants to disclose. And she's said very little.'

For the purpose of the counselling that Merle is receiving, does she actually need to have disclosed more information about her family? Does Alec need to know about other uncles, aunts, cousins, siblings, the whereabouts of her father? He could have spent much of the first session finding all this out, but what value would it have had other than information on file? Merle's issues are centred on work and on her relationship with her aunt. Yes, the relationship with her mother is a factor too, but there is not time to deal with everything. The client is trusted to bring what they need to. Family histories can tempt counsellors into becoming knowledgeable experts on their clients' lives with the power to make them better. The person-centred approach affirms the clients as the experts, and the therapeutic relationship as having the power to heal, or to unlock the client's own healing potential. The counsellor is the necessary human being to foster the presence of that relationship.

'I guess the work issues are too in her face, I mean she's working in a demanding environment, and then to have your boss on your back, it's outrageous. And I can really appreciate how difficult it is to not take sides, not get into advice giving.'

'I'm not there for that. That's available through the Human Resources department if she wants that.'

'But it sounds like your client, Merle, you say, is changing, is beginning to think differently.'

'And that's what is so encouraging, it's whether she can maintain it. And I guess I can't try and encourage that. If she slides back well, I have to help her in that place, and maybe she'll find her strength again.'

'Can't do it for her. She has to find her own way. But that can be frustrating. I'm sure I'd want to get in there and make something happen, at least part of me would, but I have to keep that contained.'

'I suppose it throws up issues for both of us when working therapeutically with these kinds of issues.'

'Sure does. Anyway, so, Merle is questioning her aunt's attitude and thinking about facing up to her boss.'

'That's right. And like I say, I'm mindful of avoiding taking sides, but I guess in a way she may well perceive me as doing that simply because talking to me is encouraging her to be different.'

'Mhmm, and it can bring up all kinds of feelings for clients, depending on how they interpret what you do, how you are.'

Alec pondered on Bernadette's last comment. Yes, he had no idea exactly how Merle would interpret how he was as a counsellor. He may not have directed her into thinking the way that she now did, or into the actions that she was now planning to take, but they had certainly emerged out of the therapeutic relationship, out of the way he was relating to her. She could end up blaming him, or blaming therapy, for making things worse, making her feel like doing things that she later regrets.

'You look very thoughtful.'

'I am. I can see how I could get blamed if it leads to a bad experience for Merle. As a person-centred counsellor I don't want to push her. In fact, I honestly don't know what is the right action to take. I mean, I know the options, but insofar as what is right for Merle at this stage, at this time in her life, in her career, I simply don't know. Though I have to say I hope she does tackle it. There are too many people in positions of power who have very suspect attitudes towards people of colour.'

'And particularly women of colour.'

'Yes, and that adds another layer to it, of course.'

'So you do have an agenda, as you say, you hope she tackles it, but you also say you don't know what's right for her at this time. Is there a contradiction there?'

'Yes, well, when you put it like that, maybe there is. But I can't deny what I think and feel, I just have to maybe ensure it doesn't cloud my responses.'

'So, putting the issue of siding with her because of her boss to one side, what about the over-compensating issue?'

'Yes, that's maybe more difficult. I don't think it's happening, but there was a time in the last session when Merle talked of being fed up being treated as just "a little black nurse", her words, and that really was powerful. And quite challenging to find the right words to empathise with. I actually used her words, but I didn't like hearing myself say them. I still don't. It's not how I see her or would want to see her, although, sure, she is little, black and she is a nurse. But you wouldn't hear people referring to themselves as being seen as a "little white nurse", so the very concept with the emphasis it has says something.'

'It's derogatory, or it can be. So the words may be descriptive, but use of those words together makes it highly likely to have a racist motivation. And it's oppressive as well, the little, yeah, and we have to be aware that there is the motivation behind the words and the way they are heard. You can get so used to it, you don't hear it – I'm talking as a black woman, here – but in reality you do hear it, you've just learned to push away the pain. But we need that pain, we need it to make us affirm who we are, what we are.' Bernadette paused with a big smile. 'See, you get me going too.'

'It's great to hear.' Alec really meant it. And he was sad that there was still the need for people to have to be fired up, had to still deal with the pain of racist attitudes, remarks and behaviours. If it made him uncomfortable what about the target? And what was he doing about it? His thoughts went back to Merle and the words that had been used.

'I don't know if anyone has said those words to her, but Merle used them to describe how she feels some people see her, or look at her.'

'It's still oppressive, the fact that she is left with that thought, yes?'

'I can see that.'

'So how would you describe her if someone, say, was to ask, what's your new client like? I mean, I know you did describe her earlier, what did you say?'

'I said she was a nurse, and I think I said struggling with issues of racism and oppression. I don't think I actually referred to her colour.'

'No, you didn't, it was implied by virtue of the issues. But if you were to describe her in terms of colour?'

'I'd say she was black, I guess.'

'So, you'd say your new client is a black nurse?'

Alec stopped as a thought struck him. 'Yes I would, but, and of course this isn't new but it's come back into the foreground, would I have said she was a white nurse if she was white, or would I just have said she's a nurse?'

Bernadette moved her head to one side and opened her hands in a gesture that Alec took to mean, 'there you go'.

'And I also want to say as well that I don't want to get so caught up in political correctness that I lose the spontaneity in my use of language.'

'Mhmm, but racial bias is very much embedded in the language we use, so freedom to be spontaneous could be a licence for racism.'

'And for me, as well as the importance of the language, there is also the meaning, the intention behind the words, the thought or feeling from which they emerge.'

'OK, I'm going to be devil's advocate here, and I'm not going to get you to do this, but maybe it's something to think about. You write down ten words that you associate with the word black. Then you write down ten words you associate with the word white. Now, when you hear someone refer, say, to a black man, a black nurse, a black boy, you're carrying a whole list of meanings, and that – and I think it's a good use of the word – and that very likely colours how you think and how you feel.'

Alec nodded.

'So, I'm working with a psychiatric nurse who lives in London.' Alec thought for a moment. 'But to not mention her colour, am I somehow at risk of not respecting an important part of her?'

'Just because you do not mention it, does that mean you do not respect it?'

'No.'

'What if someone asks you about me, what your supervisor is like. Would you mention my colour?'

'I'd mention your approach, and maybe that you are Afro-Caribbean, yes, I think I would.'

'And if I was white and lived in Hertfordshire, would you then mention my colour or race, or just that your supervisor works with such-and-such a theory and lives in Hertfordshire?'

'Yes, you're right, I very probably wouldn't mention your colour.'

'Something to think about, yes?'

'Yes. Yes, you're right. And it's all about the difficulty in seeing past the colour of someone's skin. And when and when not to highlight it.' He paused. 'Whether you say it or not, you think it and you make associations with it. Yes, how to acknowledge and respect without assumptions and prejudices that have nothing to do with the person, simply because of the colour of their skin.'

'Because it's obvious, their face is in our face, know what I mean?'

Alec smiled. Bernadette had a wonderful way of saying it as it was.

She continued. 'I don't think all of that was very person-centred, but in a way maybe it was in that it relates to your clients and I need to be true to what I think and feel about all of this. It's important to sometimes use supervision time in this way.'

'I agree, that's fine by me. The thought that is with me is around how, in time limited working, there isn't time for so much of this to emerge, but in a much longer therapeutic relationship then these kinds of issues might well be worked with in the immediacy of the relationship.'

'Sure. In a longer relationship with the counsellor seeking to be congruent in the relationship and the client working towards greater congruence, then issues of perception around race and culture, and the use of language, are likely to emerge. And certainly an experienced client – I mean someone who is quite self-aware, or who may be a therapist themselves, if they entered into a mixed-race therapeutic relationship would very likely want to clarify these kinds of issues, though not everyone might, of course.'

'In time limited work I have to be really aware of these issues, because if there isn't time to raise them and work through them, then I have to work in the knowledge of my uncertainty over my client's perception of me, whilst being as clear and open to myself about my own reactions and responses.'

'I'm going to say that in time limited work you can't afford to bring these issues into the relationship, and that sounds like you can if it is longer term. But I don't mean that. It's not appropriate but, well, not easy to avoid. Maybe what I'll say is that in time limited work maybe you have to be sharper?'

'Something like that. The time limited nature of the work makes it more focused, maybe more intense, not sure about that though, but certainly more focused.' Alec thought about what he had said.

'OK, anything else on this as we've spent a lot of time on it, which I think is helpful and it has application not just to Merle.'

'It has been useful.'

'Anything else about your work with her?'

'No, I think I need to move on to talk about other clients.'

Points for discussion

- What are your reactions to the dialogue between Alec and Bernadette? Was it an appropriate use of supervision time?

- What else could Alec have usefully brought to this supervision session?
- Were Bernadette's responses in line with person-centred principles?
- If you were Alec, what specifically would you be taking from this supervision session?
- Write notes for this supervision session as if you were Bernadette.

CHAPTER 5

Counselling session 5: client feels overwhelmed; counsellor feels disconnected

The supervision session had made a strong impression on Alec. As he sat waiting for Merle to arrive for her next counselling session, he was pondering on what impact it may have on how he would be with her. He thought that perhaps it had left him more sensitive to the uncertainties around perception and the impact of one person on another where there were visible differences of colour, culture; and also, of course, of gender. Here he was, a white man, working with a black woman on issues associated with her experience of racism and oppression from a white man. He realised that he hadn't really explored his feelings as a white man in this context in supervision. He had touched on it, but the session had moved away and he now regretted it, and had actually spent time the following evening making the lists that Bernadette had mentioned and used that as a way into his feelings.

Alec owned his discomfort as a white man. And whilst he was self-aware enough to know that the racist attitudes and behaviours that were frequently seen in the news, and thinly disguised by some political movements whilst others were quite openly racist – strange that, he thought, when inciting racial hatred was an illegal act – were those of others, he just happened to have the same colour skin. He didn't need to be personally ashamed, but he felt a certain sense of feeling oppressed into a sense of shame because his skin colour would mean that in the minds of some he was like the rest. And, yes, he did want to prove otherwise and that meant perhaps being more outwardly visible with his wish to encourage racial tolerance, respect and understanding. Strange, he thought, but like people from a particular ethnic group feeling they have to do better than white counterparts to be recognised and valued, it seemed he had to do more to feel that his non-racism was recognised and valued.

He brought his thoughts back and closed his eyes, going through his ritual to clear unwanted thoughts and feelings before the session, and to bring himself into a more sensitive place with a clearer awareness of what was present for him. When he opened his eyes it was just about time for the session, and he got up and went to see if Merle was in the waiting room.

Merle got up when she saw Alec and she followed him back to the counselling room.

'So, how do you want to use today?'

'I haven't made the list.'

Alec noticed a sense of disappointment and hoped that it hadn't shown on his
face, it could so easily be a reaction that might imply to Merle a certain dis-
approval, and he didn't feel that or want to communicate that. But he was
disappointed, and he also appreciated that, as he had said in supervision, her
new way of being was developing and, well, he didn't know the circumstances.

'Mhmm.' Alec realised it was a difficult thing to respond to. He didn't want to
direct her into an explanation with a comment that would convey a kind of
questioning as to why. He didn't want to say something like, 'fine, OK', because
very likely Merle would not be feeling it was OK or fine. He simply adopted what
he hoped was an accepting facial expression and waited to see how Merle
would continue.

'All kinds of reasons. Crazy week. Mum's been bad so my head's been in another
place. When I did find a bit of time, I don't know, I just felt like I didn't have the
energy. Feel like I've lost my way. It seemed so clear after last week, but, well,
I haven't done it.'

'So, how your mother has been, not much time or energy and a feeling that
you've kind of lost your way with it.'

'I don't know, I suppose I'm feeling like it's all too much effort, at least at the
moment.' Merle felt quite dispirited. In fact, it had been an effort to get to
the counselling appointment. She had been tempted to phone up and cancel.
It had been another crazy start to the day. It just seemed like the patients were
demanding more and more and expecting to be made better without making
the effort themselves. And she knew that wasn't fair, it was only a few, but
they were so demanding, they just seemed to dominate her diary. And she
could feel a headache coming on. She often developed them when she was
under stress. Sometimes they'd develop into a migraine. She hoped that this
one wouldn't.

'All too much at the moment, it sounds like you've had a tough week, a really
tough week.'

'Like everything happening at once. Mum makes me so mad. She gets into this
hopeless state of mind. She's had depression on and off for a number of years.
I don't think she ever really got over dad leaving, but she was like it before then.
I know she was affected by her parents dying – she was in her late twenties. They
both died young. I can remember them vaguely as a child, but not clearly. I guess
I went to my aunt as a kind of replacement, really, she was an aunt and a grandmother to me in many ways, and a mother as well at times.' Merle was thinking back to her past as she was speaking. She could remember going to stay with
friends – she wasn't allowed to go to either of her grandparents' funerals. At the
time, she didn't really know any better, but now she regretted it. Somehow not
being there left it in the air, and although at the time she wouldn't have been
thinking like that, as an adult it now seemed so important, somehow.

'So your aunt was many people to you: aunt, grandmother and mother.'

Merle nodded. 'I guess she was more important to me than anyone else.' She could feel the tears beginning to well up as she spoke. There were days when she could think of her aunt Jessie without being upset, but other days it felt as raw as it did when she had heard that she had died. It wasn't that it was unexpected. She had had heart problems for a while, and had been taken into hospital after another bout of pain in her chest. She had died during the night, quite peacefully, they had said. She had visited her that evening.

'Yes, a very important lady in your life, the most important.'

'I can still see her lying in the bed. She had her teeth out and was smiling, holding my hand. She was so thin. But her eyes, they still sparkled, but I think she knew. I don't know.' She felt the tears break over her eye-lids. She swallowed and closed her eyes, but couldn't hold back the emotions any longer. She took a tissue from the box and held it to her face, the tears continuing to flow, her own heart aching for the aunt that she would never see again.

'Important for you to have been there.'

Merle nodded. She'd wanted to be there. She'd been the last family member to see her alive, and somehow that felt right, that felt how it should have been.

'She ... told ... me,' the words came out broken between short, sharp breaths, 'that ... she ... loved ... me ..., that ... I ... was ... the ... daughter ... she'd ... never ... had.' The tears again got the better of her as another wave of emotion surged through her, causing the lump in her throat to feel even hotter. She swallowed again.

'She must have loved you dearly.'

Merle continued to sob, pausing momentarily as she reached for another, placing it over her face. Her breath was still in short gasps. 'I'm sorry.'

'No need to feel sorry. Your aunt meant so much and so many things to you. You have these feelings because you loved her.'

Merle nodded, still holding the tissue to her face. She had her hands held tight to her face, her head moving ever so slightly from side to side. Alec sat, his own heart going out to her. She stayed in that position for a couple of minutes, the waves of emotion slowly subsiding, the sobs becoming more spaced out. 'Oh dear. I feel wretched.'

'It's horrible to lose someone we love, someone so special.'

'I suppose I feel like this because of ... ' she sniffed and swallowed, ' ... because of how important she was to me.' Merle screwed up the tissue and took another, dabbing around her eyes, and then blew her nose. She took a deep breath. 'I suppose that's how it is.'

'Mhmm, that can be the price of love.'

Merle was looking down, her hands clasped tightly in her lap. 'You know, I still can't believe she's not here. I mean, I still think that maybe it was a bad dream, that I'll wake up and she'll be there and I'll be able to go and visit her again.' She smiled weakly, swallowing again as the lump in her throat felt a little larger.

> Merle does not respond to the words used by Alec. They are his words. They probably have little meaning to Merle, if they had she would very likely have acknowledged them. It isn't that what he has said is incorrect, they probably do sum up something of the relationship between losing someone you love and feeling hurt. But it's not where Merle is focused at this moment. If she had, she would probably have agreed with him. Instead, she has shifted to a focus on it all feeling like a bad dream.

Alec nodded, 'yes, as if somehow nothing has changed.'

She looked up, 'yes, as if nothing has changed.' Merle paused. 'But it has happened, and everything has changed, hasn't it?' Her face was tight-lipped.

Alec nodded again. 'Yes, everything has changed.' There wasn't anything more to say in response. He felt a mixture of sympathy and empathy for Merle. He knew from his own experience how horrible it was to lose someone who was important. He had had a close relationship with his grandfather who was a really practical man who had spent hours with him building boats and planes. It had taken him a long time, as a young man, to come to terms with his death. He had always seemed so alive, that was what had made it difficult, it had just seemed so impossible to accept that he was no more. It had always struck him how hard it was to imagine someone not existing who you had known so well. Like trying to imagine yourself dead, you can't do it. You can't imagine someone's non-existence because the moment you think about them they are back in existence in your mind, in your heart, in your memories. The only way to imagine someone not existing is to not think about them. At least, that was the conclusion he had finally come to many years later. But he still thought of his grandfather, he was still alive to him through his memories, and he still had two of the models they had made together. He smiled and then realised he'd drifted away from Merle. She was looking at him.

'Sorry, drifted into my own memories for a moment.'

'Someone special?'

Alec knew the focus was now on him, but he accepted the reality of the situation and realised he had to go with it, and facilitate the focus back on to Merle when the time was right. 'Yes, my grandfather, he was a special man. I'm sure my relationship with him was different to the one you had with your aunt, but, well, I know how it can hurt to lose someone that was important, and whose importance goes back into your childhood.'

Somehow it felt important to Merle to have heard what Alec had said. She didn't know much about him, in fact, thinking about it, she didn't know anything, other than that he was a counsellor. So hearing what he had said somehow made him a little more real, more present, more of a person, somehow. It felt like they had something in common.

> A difficult situation and yet one that can have therapeutic value as shown by Merle's inner response to what Alec has said. However, one difficulty

could be that the client makes the assumption that the counsellor under-stands what it is like to lose her aunt, and that can discourage the client from exploring it further because she doesn't feel she needs to tell the coun-sellor; he already knows. This then cuts across the therapeutic need for the client to describe what she needs to have heard. Or does it? Does the fact that a self-disclosure is taken to mean, by the client, that the counsellor under-stands, actually have a positive therapeutic impact? It's not that a counsel-lor would want to try and convey directly that they understand what a client is experiencing because of what they have experienced; although in this instance Alec has said that he knows 'how it can hurt to lose someone that was important, and whose importance goes back into your childhood'. This may have gone too far, but as is ever the case in therapy, it is down to how the client internalises and interprets what has been said. Maybe, in a particular therapeutic relationship, such a disclosure will prove helpful, whilst in another it will be less so. Maybe, too, Alec's earlier comment about the price of love can be seen as emerging from his own loss, not as a result of his feeling connected to Merle in her acknowledgement of loss.

'Good to hear something about you.' Yes it was, but then she felt the psychiatric nurse in her emerging. She wanted to say something more to Alec, but it felt wrong, somehow. That wasn't why she was there. She felt herself frown.

'I see you're frowning. Maybe I took the focus away from you.'

'No, I just felt myself wanting to go into "psychiatric-nurse" mode then. And then I didn't want to.'

'Towards me, do you mean?'

Merle nodded.

'I guess that's a big part of you, but not the part you want to bring here, at least, not at the moment.'

'No, I don't. I appreciate what you just said. It isn't easy.'

'No. And you were with your aunt, telling me how you were the last family member to spend time with her before she died. That must have been so impor-tant to you.'

Merle nodded, 'yes, it was'. But she felt distant from that experience now. Like she had lost her focus. She felt unsure, uneasy, as if she had been pulled away, out of herself, but not placed back down anywhere in particular.

Alec felt disconnected from Merle, not that he had been necessarily aware of being connected, but suddenly things felt different, awkward. He could only put it down to his self-disclosure following his own drift into his past. 'I feel as though I'm disconnected. It's me, I think what I said has really disturbed the place where we were when you had been talking about being with your aunt and how much she meant to you.'

Merle was moving back to her memories of her aunt. Yes, she had felt pulled away from it, but it felt as though it was coming back. 'There's something about people who feel so alive to us, and who then are suddenly not there. I don't know, I suppose it's just so hard to accept, I mean really accept, deep down accept.'

Alec nodded, 'you mean hard to really deep down accept that they've gone.'

'It's like they haven't, not really, they're still with you, in your memories. I can still see her, and hear her voice. Suppose it fades, voices that is, but the image is clear. Do you find that?'

Alec realised that the dialogue had shifted, it was now much more of a conversation. Well, maybe that was how it needed to be, but he also wondered if that was a bit of a cop out on his part. He shouldn't have drifted, and maybe then he shouldn't have self-disclosed, but he did, and he would need to explore it in supervision. Meanwhile, he had to go with the session as it was now focused, what else was there to do? Merle was seeking feedback from him. He felt he should respond.

'The voice fades, and to some degree so do the memories. Photos keep them alive, but that's me and you may have a very different experience.'

'I've got photos, but I want to have memories that are active. There are videos at home of me and my brother when we were much younger, and auntie Jessie is on some of those. They're going to be important.' Merle stopped speaking as she recalled the conversation she had with her aunt that last evening.

'Mhmm, it will help to keep her memory alive.'

There are times when therapeutic dialogue does take on more of a conversational tone, and it can play a part. But it is about appropriateness and whether it is therapeutically helpful for the client. The person-centred counsellor will acknowledge and accept a client's need to experience a more conversational exchange, and will perhaps go with that, though they might also acknowledge it at some point if that feels right related to whatever is being explored.

Sometimes it is very difficult to maintain a 'counselling dialogue' for a complete session; counsellor and client can feel the need to have some relief from it. However, that is not a reason for counsellors to simply chat to their clients, and certainly not to impose a more conversational tone which can have the effect of causing a client to avoid difficult areas which may be induced so the counsellor can avoid their own discomfort.

Merle could hear her aunt's voice. 'You know, that evening in the hospital, she knew she was dying. I suppose I probably did as well though I wasn't letting myself think about it, but she was lying there, holding my hand, and she looked at me, it was such a searching look. "You take care of yourself, little Merle, everything'll be alright, you'll see. Have faith. You're doing the Lord's work. It's what's in your heart that matters, my dear. That's all He's interested in." She squeezed my hand and smiled at me.' The emotions were present again. 'I guess I am doing the Lord's work, going amongst the sick, caring, trying to help. I don't really think of it that way much, it's what I do, what I want to do. But the way she said it, I'll never forget the words. They seemed to command attention. She seemed so frail and yet her voice was strong, or so it seemed.' Merle took another deep breath.

'A very profound message.'

'Makes me feel quite still talking about it. I can feel the emotion, but also a stillness.' She shook her head. 'That's what matters. That's what really matters. What's in here.' She put her right hand over her heart. 'She's right, isn't she?' Merle paused, and continued, 'I think she's right. It's about how much you care about people, how much you put their needs first. That's what I want to do, but it's so hard when everyone wants so much, and you feel so exhausted by it all.' Merle's thoughts were back to the unit, to her patients, to the demands made upon her. How she wanted to live up to the ideal of being able to keep giving. But she knew she couldn't as well, it was too much, all too much at times.

'It's the ideal, what you strive for, but it's so hard when the demand is greater than what you are able to give.'

'There are so many people, they need time, time to make sense of themselves, of their lives, and we just don't have the time to give to them. We really don't. We try, and we do help people, but not enough. And here am I wanting to really rock the boat. I mean, oh I don't know. This idea of complaining to my boss, taking out a grievance, what good will it do? It'll cause trouble and I don't need that.'

'Mhmm it feels like complaining to your boss, or taking out a grievance, is just going to cause trouble, trouble you feel you don't need at the moment.'

The counsellor maintains empathy and does not slip into trying to encourage the client to do something. He acknowledges what he has heard the client say, no more, allowing her to move on without her focus or thinking being distracted by anything from him.

Merle sat quietly for a moment, thinking about what she had said. 'And hearing you say that back to me, I know as well that maybe I owe it to myself, and maybe others, to say or do something. But today, now, at the moment, it seems too much. Maybe next week, maybe I'll feel different, but just at the moment it all seems too much.'

'You don't have to do anything that you don't feel you want to.'

'Yes, I know. I suppose I don't know what I want.' She paused. 'No, I do know. I want a quiet life and time to do the work that I want to do, time to really help my patients, time to make a difference and not feel as though I am on a kind of, what do they call it, treadmill. Patients come in, move through and go out, and we have to keep up with them. Maybe it's more like a conveyer belt and we run beside it. And it's getting faster and more people are coming through, and some of them maybe shouldn't be on the mental health conveyer belt but there's nowhere else for them to go, so that's where they get put, and we have to respond, react, make them safe.' Her voice had speeded up. She shook her head. 'Maybe it's me. Maybe I'm weak. Maybe I can't do the work.'

'That how it feels, that you're weak and aren't any good at what you do?'

Merle sat quietly considering what she had just said. She knew it wasn't true. 'No, no it's just that sometimes I doubt myself.'

'And now is one of those times?'

'But something has to change. I can't go on like this. I've booked some time out, by the way, I should have mentioned it. I'm off next week, maybe that'll give me some time to think and get some energy back. I'm off with a friend to a Greek Island for a week; get away from it all. Not one of the busy ones, a small island with beaches and sun and time to just forget about it all.'

'Sounds good and sounds really important. Give yourself time to get some energy back and think about things.'

'I need it.' She paused. 'So, I won't be around until the following week.'

Alec checked his diary. 'That's fine. Same time, same day?'

'Yes please. How many sessions will that be?'

'It will be, let me just check, er, it will be the sixth, but you cancelled one, so it will be your fifth session.'

'So I'm half way. Half way to somewhere. Is this what counselling is like?'

'People have different experiences, but it usually makes people connect with feelings, think about things, it's not always easy.'

'Tell me about it!' Merle checked the time. 'Time to go. I've given myself a bit of time this week to relax, haven't booked anyone in for an hour, so I'm going to have a leisurely coffee break and read a magazine in that new coffee shop round the corner.'

'Give yourself a treat. You've earned it, I think.'

'Thanks. So, see you in two weeks.'

'Yes, have a great time away and give yourself a bit of a break from thinking about work.'

'I'll try, but I feel I need to do some serious thinking as well.'

Merle headed out of the door. She felt easier than she had when she had arrived. Yes, she was looking forward to her holiday, it was certainly overdue. She'd give it all more thought. She still had mixed feelings, but she was also feeling more certain that she couldn't carry on with things as they were. When she had described it like a conveyer belt, it really had made an impression on her. And she didn't want it to be like that. She did feel that anyone who was particularly complex seemed to be detailed to her. Maybe she was too good at her job, but other people were capable and experienced, not just her. Oh, she didn't know, and she didn't want to think about it. She wanted her coffee, and probably a large piece of cake as well, what the hell, and make a bit of time for herself.

Alec, meanwhile, was writing up his notes. He was very concerned that he had drifted off in the session. That was very unusual and he knew he had to talk it through with Bernadette when he next saw her. What had he been thinking of? He tried to recall what had happened. Merle had been talking about her aunt in hospital, how special she was, or something like that, and he'd gone, drifted off. Why then? She'd talked of her aunt at other times, but it hadn't triggered him into thinking of his grandfather. What was different this time? He thought about it some more. What had been different, what had she said? He caught his breath. Yes, yes, of course, so obvious, but why hadn't he immediately realised it? He remembered how he'd woken up one morning and for some reason thought his grandfather was still alive. He'd had a really vivid dream about him, and he really thought he was alive. He'd said something to his parents about going and visiting granddad, and they'd both looked at him somewhat astonished. He remembered them looking at each other, as if neither knew what to say. It was his father who had responded. 'Alec, are you OK? Don't you remember, your granddad is dead. Don't you remember going to his house, seeing how everything had changed?' How everything had changed. He took a deep breath. He felt his own emotions rising. He needed to have a break, and a cup of coffee himself, and get himself ready for his next client.

Points for discussion

- Evaluate the quality of Alec's congruence in this session.
- How did Alec communicate unconditional positive regard?
- Would you have handled Alec's disconnection differently if you had been him?
- With regard to Merle's indecision as to what to do, explain the process in terms of person-centred theory.
- What feelings does the session leave you with? Other than the connection made to his grandfather, what else might Alec take to supervision?
- Write notes for this session.

CHAPTER 6

Counselling session 6: a fresh determination

Merle spent the first half of the session talking about the holiday she had been on and how she had decided that she was going to say something at work. Being free of it all for a few days had given her a chance to think clearly, and her friend had been really supportive and encouraging. She had written down the incidents when she felt she was treated unfairly and had already told her manager that she wanted to speak to him. They'd booked a time on the day after her counselling session. She'd felt anxious but determined to see it through.

'I guess it was having a bit of free space to really reflect and think it through. It's been so hectic, I haven't really had time to think, not clearly, not with so much else swirling around.'

'So having that space was really helpful, your mind was a little more freed up.'

'Yes, it really did feel like a break, a real break. I remember thinking, as the plane took off, leave it behind, leave it all on the runway. Let it go. And I did. The first half of the week I really did devote myself to being on holiday, and then I felt, OK, now let's give it some thought. So, I came back, determined and ready to have my say.'

Alec nodded.

'It was Kathy, my friend, who made a particularly interesting comment. She said that a friend had told her a while back, "you know when you need to change something when that something starts to make you unwell". It has been making me unwell. I haven't felt like me, particularly the last year. It does feel harder to keep going. And maybe my boss changing his attitude won't change things enough, maybe the job is simply too exhausting, too demanding, I don't know. If that is the case, then I'll think again, but for now I need to say my piece.'

Alec nodded again. He felt good about what Merle was saying. She sounded like she really was owning her decision. Clearly her friend had played a part in encouraging her to make her decision, well, that's what friends are for. In a way he saw the counselling as having prepared the ground, but like ploughing things up, preparing the soil ready for the seed of some new idea or action to be sown. He genuinely felt warmth for Merle in her struggle to make choices and decisions that were right for her. It was good to see. So many people put up with things, he'd done it himself, not saying anything, making the best of it, when

actually something needed to change, needed to give. He knew how organisations could just carry on in their own way, maintaining their own cultures
until or unless someone spoke up and forced an issue on to the agenda, and
even then it could take a lot of pushing for change to occur. The NHS, whilst it
is broken up into trusts and primary care teams, is still a vast organisation with
its own culture. It can take time for new directions to take hold.
The presence of oppression and racism was not new to him. They were problems,
not affecting everyone, but those who were often found their careers suppressed
and their general well-being undermined. He had seen people badly damaged.
Often, staff who were bullied, had had similar experiences elsewhere, though
that was not necessarily always the case. But it could and did affect a person's
self-concept, causing them to believe that they only deserved second best,
that there was no point in trying to change anything, or that somehow it was
their fault and that they attracted that kind of behaviour towards themselves.

The truth, however, is that bullying in the NHS, or any other, workplace is
unacceptable and is damaging to the target. For Alec, one of the attractions
of the person-centred approach is the way that it is rooted in a philosophy
that encourages a more equal power balance. It is an approach that has
application in management as well as therapy. He wished a few more managers would adopt it. Management is about relationship and the principles
of the person-centred approach could help encourage the best from people,
and a more collaborative atmosphere.

'So, you say you're meeting the team manager tomorrow.'
'I'm not going to attack him, but I just want to give him my view of what has been
happening, how I feel unfairly treated, and that I want him to take seriously
what I am saying. I don't want to come across as threatening, but I do want
him to know that whilst I'm not taking out a grievance at this stage, I will do
if I feel that the situation continues.'
'You sound very calm and clear as you are speaking, it feels to me that you have
really owned what you need to do.'
'That's good to hear. Yes. I think that's what has changed, what going away has
done. It has helped me step back and then get hold of what I know I need to do.
I've got my life to lead and I want to get on with it. I don't want work to be such
a problem. I want a healthy working life, that's the bottom line, I just want to
feel that I have a healthy working life.'
Alec thought of the phrase Merle had used and it reminded him of the 'Improving
Working Lives' initiatives that were being introduced in NHS trusts.

'Improving Working Lives' is an initiative to enhance working environments and ensure needs, ideas and concerns are communicated between
staff and managers. It includes good human resources practice and policy

(including equality and diversity issues), initiatives such as flexible working, child-care facilities or arrangements for staff members, reduced membership fees at health clubs and gyms, and staff having a voice in the organisation.

'Yes, a healthy working life. That's quite a powerful statement.'

'I think sitting on the beach in the sun, and just the whole relaxed environment made me think, really think, about how life could be. I mean, I know it can't be quite like that, but the contrast between that and the frantic activity, the rushing around, the stress, all of it, I could somehow see it for what it was – utter madness. No time to think, to reflect on your practice. It's not healthy, it really isn't.' Merle shook her head. 'Sitting there just thinking about work I could feel the tension coming back. But you get used to it, you don't realise just how tense you have become.'

'Being there, being away from it, made you realise how much tension you had been carrying.'

'And I had a massage whilst I was away, there was a massage service at the hotel. Was that painful! In my back and my shoulders; again it made me aware of just how tense I'd become. I've decided to continue with that, I am going to find somewhere locally. I need to look after myself.'

'Yes, make healthy choices and look after yourself.' Alec kept his response brief to allow Merle to continue with the flow. Realising her need to look after herself, after her health, was clearly now important to her. It was clearly a key element in her decision to make changes in her life and in her work.

'And I'm going to take my full lunch breaks, and I'm going to have short breaks during the day. The smokers go out for cigarette breaks, so I shall have fresh-air breaks.'

'You sound really strong, really clear and determined. Lunch breaks and fresh-air breaks.'

'I have to. I've changed. It's like I've suddenly got to see things differently. I needed that space away. And coming here. I think the timing was right. Part of me had had enough but was too exhausted to really do anything about it. But going away helped me get a fresh perspective and my energy back. Seeing you had sort of stirred things up, I guess, made me more aware, but I needed that time and that space, and the energy, to realise what I had to do, and to feel that I could do it.'

'So the timing was right, the counselling stirred things up and the holiday gave you time to reflect, get a clearer view and energy to act.'

'Now I just have to do it!' Merle grinned through tight lips.

'Yes, making it all happen.'

'But that's down to me, at least to begin with, and then we'll see how others react.' She was thinking of her team leader, wondering how he would react. Surely he'd listen. He had to. 'And I'm not going to give my manager a lot of time, either. I need to maintain momentum. If he's unhelpful, unreasonable or doesn't accept what I have to say, then I'll put in a formal grievance. I feel I have to whilst I have the energy. I know what it's like. If I'm not careful I'll end up back as I was feeling a couple of weeks back, really unsure as to what to do and whether I could do it.'

'You're aware that you need to keep the momentum up. You don't want to feel overwhelmed or feel like you did before.'

No, Merle thought, no, I have to avoid that.

The session drew to a close. Merle had talked through with her friend what she was going to say to her boss, and she didn't feel she needed to go over that with Alec. She felt she had said enough about it, and just wanted to get it over with. Alec wished her well with her meeting and she thanked him. They agreed the next session would be the following week.

Counselling session 7: difference and diversity

Alec had been wondering how things had worked out for Merle. She had seemed so fired up and clear the previous week, but he appreciated, as well, how this could get lost when things began to get too much. As she sat down in the counselling room, he looked across. She seemed somehow quite purposeful in the way she had hung up her coat and was sitting down.

'So, where do you want to begin this week?'

'I've put a grievance in writing. He wasn't very receptive, I didn't think. Yes, he said he was concerned, but it was the way he spoke, he didn't seem at all genuine, felt like he was just trying to calm me down, tell me that I was imagining things. It wasn't that he said it directly, but it was the way he spoke. He said, "I'm sorry you feel that way," and "I'm sorry you see it like that." Always about how I saw it, not how it is.' Merle looked over towards Alec as she spoke, she looked angry.

'I can see the anger. He wasn't going to accept what you were saying so you're taking it further.'

'I am, and that's how it is.' She tossed back her hair. 'I'm sorry it has become the way it has, I don't think it needed to, but I've done it now and I have a meeting with the service manager and someone from human resources coming up. They want to hear what I have to say. I gather they are also going to meet up with my boss.'

'So you have this meeting and it will give you an opportunity to explain what has been happening.'

'And he's been a bit quieter the last couple of days. I don't think he thought I'd take it this far. But he was wrong. I've changed, well, I'm changing.'

'Yes, and it seems as though you are maintaining your resolve.'

'Most of the time. I do feel doubt and anxiety as well, you know, wondering if I'm just going to make it worse for myself in the long run.'

Alec nodded, 'doubting and anxious as to what will happen long-term.'

'I mean, if I'm still at the unit with him, we still have to work together, you know? But at least he'll be under the spotlight a bit, at least, I hope so. I've only met the service manager a couple of times, usually when she has come to meetings. She seemed nice enough, but, well, you don't know, do you?'

'You're not sure how much you can trust the way she will handle the grievance process, do you mean?'

Merle had looked away, she was feeling uncertain again. It came and went. It usually got worse when she thought about how things would be afterwards. She didn't want more hassle, the problem was she couldn't actually imagine her boss being different. That was the real problem. If she could imagine him being fairer, and being more approachable, then maybe she would feel differently. But she couldn't.

'I just wish I didn't have to go through all of this, that I could just get on with my work and feel that the work was distributed fairly and that the demands made on me were realistic. That's all I want. Is that too much?'

'Sounds very reasonable, to want to be given a fair amount of work and time to do it.' Alec was aware of knowing how he'd heard similar summaries from other staff over the years.

'He started going on about Agenda for Change, telling me that it would all be different, that I would be assessed as to my competence for the job and that I'd better measure up.' Merle shook her head. 'I wavered when he said that, I could feel my voice get wobbly, but I remembered what a friend had said who had been to a presentation about it recently. She'd explained how there were going to be job descriptions with graded competencies established for each nursing grade across the Trust, except in some specific areas where jobs had unique responsibilities, and that the assessment for competence would involve other members of staff trained in the process. That it wasn't just up to the manager. I remembered that and found my determination again. Told him that he might think that was how Agenda for Change worked, but I knew different. And then I pointed out that it was a pity he hadn't invited someone to our team to explain about Agenda for Change, which I knew had happened elsewhere. He told me he didn't see the need, and that it would happen in good time.'

'So you waivered but fortunately what you knew about Agenda for Change meant you could stand up to what he was saying.'

'I felt good about that, but it was horrible at the time. Anyway, he's got it coming to him now. But I still can't help worrying about the future.'

'Seems as though that is your main concern at the moment, what will happen after this process.' Alec felt the concern in himself and yet he also knew that the more senior managers in the Trust were keen to root out bad management and particularly confront oppression, bullying and racism. There were enough posters around declaring 'zero-tolerance', and yet it still happened. People who were on the receiving end could be made to feel vulnerable and powerless. So often it was people who had already generated a part of themselves that felt this way who were most susceptible, though not always. For others this part of their self-structure would develop in response to the negative and oppressive behaviour that they experienced towards themselves.

An area of person-centred theory that has application here is the notion of 'configuration within self'. Mearns (1999; 2000) has written about the concept of 'configurations of self'. He writes that 'a "configuration" is a hypothetical construct denoting a coherent pattern of feelings, thoughts and preferred behavioural responses symbolised or pre-symbolised by the person as reflective of a dimension of existence within the self' (Mearns, 2000, p. 102).

Patterns of feelings, thoughts and behaviour might be thought of as clustering together in association with a particular aspect of the person's felt existence. So, for instance, the person who feels oppressed or bullied, if this is an experience that they have had on a number of occasions, may develop a set of reactions to this experience. They might conceptualise it as 'victimised me' and when something happens that takes them into this particular sense of self then the associated feelings, thoughts and behaviours they have developed when they have this experience are likely to emerge and be lived out. So 'victimised me' might leave the person feeling disempowered, or thinking they are worthless or behaving in a manner that provokes further rejection in order for that part to grow and maintain its existence.

Mearns suggests that 'the self is comprised of a number of "parts" or "configurations" interrelating like a family, with an individual variety of dynamics. When the interrelationship of configurations changes, it is not that we are left with something entirely new: we have the same "parts" as before, but some which may have been subservient before are stronger, others which were judged adversely are accepted, some which were in self-negating conflict have come to respect each other, and overall the parts have achieved constructive integration with the energy release which arises from such fusion' (Mearns, 1999, pp. 147–8).

Added to this, new configurations may develop when a person is exposed to new, and repetitive, experiences. Hence someone not previously affected by bullying may, when they are, develop a bullied or victimised sense of self or configuration. Racism will also encourage the development of configurations as well, which will be linked in different ways to the person's already developed view of themselves.

As well as an individual developing configurations of self in response to being the victim of racist attitudes, we might speculate that perhaps in some way the same process may occur across a society, a kind of 'collective configuration'. It may in some way draw people together who have within themselves similar configurations. This might be another way of explaining, psychologically, the emergence of mass movements and the persistence of certain attitudes within societies. Such collective configurations, if they exist, will be true for the racist and for the victims of racism.

'Part of me feels like I don't want this to be happening, almost questioning whether I'm right, whether I should be doing what I am doing, but that part is weaker now, most of the time anyway. I think it was stronger in the past. I really felt like I had no voice, that I had to accept it, that was how it was. You got on with it, you know?'

Alec nodded. 'Part of you felt you had to accept it and get on with it, but that part is weaker now.'

'But it makes me think. We were talking about this on holiday. I mean, I was brought up here, I know my way around, but even then, I still felt trapped and powerless at times. What about all the nurses coming over from overseas now, who are new to Britain, new to the NHS, they're potentially so vulnerable, and it worries me. We don't see so many people coming over like that in mental health nursing, not as much as general nursing.' She shook her head. 'It really does make you wonder what will happen, is happening.'

Alec was aware of having had similar feelings, particularly where possible oppressed people were being brought into organisations where perhaps there might be oppressive attitudes already in existence. He hoped it wasn't as bad as he imagined it could be, but he did wonder. He had not worked for a general hospital trust, so he did not know, but the way Merle was speaking it was certainly heightening his sense of concern.

'Yes, it is a concern, a real concern, and you wonder how much people appreciate the potential difficulties. You know how difficult it was for you, in spite of your familiarity with society here.'

Merle paused. 'Somehow what I'm doing takes on a different meaning. I'm not only doing it for me, am I?'

'That how it feels, you're not only doing it for you?'

'Well, I mean, at the start, yes I was, but these kind of thoughts, you know, when you think about it, I mean, it's only by people standing up and saying no to what is unacceptable, it's the only way there will be change. If I don't shout, senior managers may never know what's happening.'

Alec nodded, although he was very much in favour of senior managers spending time in their units, getting a feel for how they work, meeting people more informally to help them get a sense of the prevailing culture, the difficulties and concerns, as well as the strengths and the opportunities that were present.

'So, it feels as though you are not only taking action for yourself, but for others as well, to make sure the senior people are more aware of what is happening?'

Merle nodded herself, slowly and thoughtfully. 'It's not good enough, is it, just letting things go?'

By connecting with her own thoughts and feelings on a personal level, Merle now connects with a kind of collective identity, realising that her voice needs to be heard not just for herself, but for everyone. This process of identifying the meeting of ones' own needs with a greater process is not unusual. Where an organisation has problems it does need people to feel empowered

> to take action, which may simply be to point out what is going on. And given that people are seeking more satisfying experiences in their lives, feeling empowered, feeling heard, feeling that they have made a positive difference and can see and feel the results, is enormously attractive. This is why counselling has a certain revolutionary edge to it, for it helps people to get in touch with themselves, it helps them to find their personal power.

'You really question whether doing nothing is good enough.'

'And that makes me feel bad because that was what I had been doing. And yet I felt that was how it had to be. I mean, yes, I thought about it, about how unfair it was, and that I wanted it to be different, but I couldn't make that jump to accepting I had to take action, or do something. I just wasn't there.' As she spoke she realised how frustrated she was with herself now, but also how sobering a thought it was, that she could be trapped by her own sense of powerlessness in a situation where there were mechanisms available to exercise power. But she couldn't, didn't, it just seemed something beyond her thinking at the time. And how many other people felt like she did, now, not just in the NHS, it wasn't fair to single it out, but in any public or private organisation. How many people – and not just those who were experiencing racial oppression, gender, sexual, disability, yes, even the way people looked, could all be used by others to oppress, leaving the victim helpless.

'Bullying just seems to be part of life. The NHS workplace, or any workplace – is it that much different from the schoolyard? I mean, is it? Same kinds of processes, just older people.'

'Living out the same attitudes and values, you mean?'

'Anyone who is different, who doesn't "go with the crowd" is at risk. It's awful. Makes me even more determined to do my bit.'

The London Hazards Centre's website 'Bullying at Work' factsheet contains the following:

'Bullying at work is any form of behaviour which is offensive, intimidating, malicious or insulting or is an abuse or misuse of power intended to undermine, humiliate, denigrate or injure individuals or groups.

'Bullying leads to *stress* and then to illness and behavioural problems if prolonged. A very high proportion of people subjected to bullying change their job as a result.

'Bullying is widespread at work. A survey by UNISON revealed that 66 per cent of the respondents had experienced or witnessed bullying. Thirty-four per cent of those bullied reported that it had gone on for more than three years.

'In over 80 per cent of cases, the bully was a manager. In almost all cases the higher management knew what was going on but did nothing about it.

'Bullying can take many forms:

- direct verbal and physical threats
- unfair use of disciplinary and assessment procedures
- blocking access to promotion, training, overtime, etc.
- setting impossible deadlines and targets
- withholding information essential to do the job properly
- excessively tight supervision
- public humiliation, including being shouted at
- persistent and undue criticism including inaccurate accusations about quality of work
- undermining responsibility
- abusive references to age, sex, race, disability or other personal characteristics
- spreading malicious rumours
- physical isolation from other workers.

'Bullying is not just an interaction between individuals; there are organisational factors at work which can facilitate it. Among these are:

- an extremely competitive environment
- fear of redundancy, cuts or reorganisation
- little participation in decision making
- poor training
- deskilling
- no clear policies or codes of conduct
- poor procedures for resolving grievances and problems
- indifferent attitude of higher management towards behaviour by front-line managers' (London Hazard Centre, 1999).

'You're finding your voice and now you want it heard.' Alec used his own metaphor but felt that it would convey to Merle what he was experiencing as happening.

'I am. I do.' She paused. 'And you know, maybe my aunt's attitude was right for her generation, maybe it was, I don't know. I still struggle with that. I mean, that attitude in the 1960s in America and, well, you wouldn't have had a civil rights movement. People had put up with it for too long and were saying "no". Yet it still goes on, maybe not as extreme, but, well, people are still getting killed because of their colour or their race. No, I don't want to say killed, murdered, that's the right word for it. Black, brown and white. But black people are more likely to be imprisoned – look at the number of black people in US prisons. I read an article about the number of black people on death row, and how suspect a lot of the sentencing is, in fact DNA evidence is being destroyed to ensure it doesn't come to light. Can you believe it? Is it any better over here? I hope so, but ...' She shook her head.

Alec was seeing a new Merle, and he didn't mean that in a patronising kind of way. He was seeing a woman, yes, a black woman – he thought of his supervision session with Bernadette – who was no longer going to accept racial oppression. He could see the fire in her eyes, the outrage that was not there when he had first met her. Then she had seemed so flat, so unable to find strength to fight back, all she could do was keep herself going at work. Now, the phrase was back with him from that earlier session, now everything had changed, was changing. He suspected that Merle might not now be able to go back to the person that she had been, and he felt good about that, and the hope that he had played a part in it in some significant, or even insignificant, way.

He didn't see much need to say a great deal, Merle was saying what needed to be said. He simply needed to let her know that he heard and understood what she was saying. 'These injustices, they really are affecting you now in a new way, black people being treated differently, badly.'

'Must be different for you, being white.'

'Yes, it is different, being white. Part of me wants to think more of myself as a human being among human beings, and though I take pride in my cultural and ethnic background, I don't want that difference to be a barrier. But I also know that when a group of people feel oppressed they will seek to strengthen their cultural identity, which is great, but somehow the risk is that it exaggerates the differences and then you are at risk of creating walls and barriers, perhaps.'

Merle nodded. 'I think you are right. I'm never too sure if Britain is really multi-cultural, not really, truly. We have a lot of diversity of ethnicity and culture, but there is a kind of invisible sense of separation, and sometimes it's all too visible. I just want to be me, you know? I'm British but I have an ethnic heritage as well. I suppose in a way I am a multi-cultural person because I kind of feel both. But some people want to be either one or the other and I'm not sure whether that just creates problems. A friend said to me a while back, ''you know, with all the inter-racial relationships, and children of mixed race, in a few generations there won't be white or black or brown, but we'll all be the same colour and that'll put an end to racism''.'

Alec smiled. He wondered. Would it? Human beings seemed to have this capacity to differentiate and separate. He hoped that one day that prevailing sense of separateness would diminish. He knew it would be a better world. But the world as it was needed to be addressed.

'All one colour.'

Merle thought about it, and although she had shared her friend's comment, she wasn't too sure whether she agreed with it. 'But I like my colour. I like the difference, it's the attitudes I don't like.'

'Yeah. You like your colour but not the racist attitudes towards you that exist because of that outward difference.'

The focus of the session moved back to Merle's determination to be heard, and then on to how she hoped her career would develop in the future. Alec noted that she seemed more able to look ahead, or was that a misapprehension on his part? Merle had thought about it and agreed that, yes, she was looking ahead more, and yes, that was worrying with the grievance and her manager, but that was short term. So, yes, maybe she was, maybe she could now think further than coping with the next day which she realised was how it had become.

Points for discussion

- Where has this session left your thoughts and feelings? What would you now need to process before seeing your next client?
- Evaluate Alec's empathic sensitivity in this session. How facilitative were his responses in enabling Merle to clarify her thoughts and feelings?
- What issues would you be taking to supervision from this session?
- What are your opinions with regard to the impact of racial difference and racism on the individual and on society?
- Write down what you understand by the term 'configuration within the self'. What attitudes, thoughts, feelings and behaviours do you feel have clustered within your own self-structure?
- Write notes for this session.

CHAPTER 7

Counselling session 8: conversational counselling

'So, all in all, it was really useful.' Merle had been telling Alec about the grievance interview she had had with the service manager and the human resources advisor. It was now half way through their session. 'As I say, they were really very concerned and quite supportive of me. They pointed out that they needed to be impartial, they were undertaking an investigation, but I felt heard, I felt taken seriously, and they seemed genuinely determined to confront issues of racism and oppression. They explained that they couldn't be sure that the events that concerned me were specifically racially motivated, and I agreed. I wasn't sure whether it was racism. I'm still not completely sure but, well, when you're black it's such a commonplace thing that you naturally assume it is racially motivated. No, I thought they were fair. They certainly said that the allegations that I had made were significant and, if true, then they would be taking the matter forward with the utmost seriousness.'

Merle was sitting back in the chair, feeling positive and relaxed, more so than she had in any previous counselling session. She wasn't sure why. Maybe it was something about feeling heard, feeling respected. Maybe it made her feel different, more confident somehow. At least, that was the conclusion she had drawn, and she realised that a lot of this was due to Alec's attitude. She felt she wanted to say something to him.

Alec was responding to what Merle had been saying, wanting to let her know that he had heard what she had been saying. 'So, all in all, it went well, you felt heard, taken seriously, and I guess glad that that part is over.'

Merle nodded. 'Yes, and I was just thinking, you know, I really couldn't have done this without coming to see you. I mean, I don't know, I've been thinking about this counselling more this past week, more than previously I suppose, but I can see that it really has helped, even though I've been confused and tearful at times, and, well, I suppose I've really not been too sure what it's been all about.'

'Yes, well, we've covered – you've covered – a lot of ground. A lot of issues over recent weeks, and I've been glad to be able to offer you time and space to talk about, feel, think, explore; be how you've needed to be.'

'It's not just the space. I mean, that's been important, and that coupled with the holiday, really helped me to appreciate the need to take time to reflect, and gave me the opportunity. It's been quite intense in some of the sessions, and whilst I have been thinking about things, I think it was going away that really gave me time, really helped me to just, I don't know, take stock of the situation. I was too close to it all, to everything that was going on before, I couldn't step back. But when I did, and having Kathy with me helped, no doubt about that, well, then I began to see things more clearly and feel more assured of what I needed to do, I guess.'

'So, it was a case of right timing, and you've made good use of it.'

'Yes, but what I was wanting to say was that it isn't just about having time or space, though that's been important. It's about having someone listen to me, take me seriously, I really mean that. To begin with I really didn't know if anyone would believe me. I didn't feel confident. I just felt in a mess, too much stuff in my head, too many feelings swirling around. But you listened. And – and this is important, and perhaps more so than I thought, certainly at first – but it is important that you are a white man. I think that had you been a white woman it would have been different, or a black woman or a black man, but you're a white man and that means I am being taken seriously by both a man, and a person who is white. And yet, if I'd had a choice at the start I would probably have asked for a black, female counsellor, and I'm sure that would have been helpful, and it would have been different.'

Differences between client and counsellor will affect the content of the counselling sessions, there can be no doubt about that. When you begin to try to make the judgement as to which mix may be right, or wrong, better or worse, for a given person or issue, you step into a very uncertain area. Who is to say? As in this example, the client may have preferred a black, female counsellor; but a white, male counsellor has had an important role in facilitating change. Would the changes have occurred whoever it was? Was the client simply on the verge of change and just needed a counsellor of any colour or gender to offer her the core conditions for the shift to occur?

As in life, we have to work with what comes our way. Sometimes we have to trust a greater process. Some may call it chance, but others may see a purpose working out, as if clients attract, or are attracted to, in some mysterious way, the counsellor they need. Except that counselling relationships can also go wrong, and the fact that there are a steady flow of counsellors from all theoretical persuasions who are adjudged to have transgressed codes of practice and ethical frameworks is testimony to this.

What we can say is that the coming into contact and relationship of two people, one called a client, one called a counsellor, where there is incongruence in the client, and there is an attempt on the part of the counsellor to communicate empathic understanding, unconditional positive regard and congruence, all of which are received by the client; then there is opportunity for constructive personality change within the client and, I think it is fair to argue, within the counsellor as well. Perhaps, where these factors are present, in some mysterious way the gender, colour, sexual orientation or any other factor of difference on the part of the counsellor does not actually matter. The conditions for constructive personality change in some sense transcend these factors. If so, then we must conclude that the philosophy of the person-centred approach genuinely has global application. Perhaps it provides the basis for not only constructive personality change, but also constructive human relationship.

'I appreciate what you say, and I actually think it's a very courageous perspective. I think, yes, it would have been different if there had been a different gender or racial mix, but whether it would have been better or not, who knows? All we have is the experience that we have and, for you, it would seem that it has proved extremely helpful. And I am sure working with a black, female counsellor would probably offer other areas of emphasis, or maybe be facilitative for you in other ways.'

'And maybe I'll try that in the future as well! I've actually realised I have a lot of respect for counselling.'

Alec smiled. It was good to hear.

Merle began speaking again. 'Yes, it's something we could do with more of in mental health. I'd like to see people being given real therapeutic time, free of the key working responsibilities – there's no doubt that it does get in the way. Clients want you to perhaps argue for them to change their medication, or be an advocate for them at a CPA (Care Programme Approach) meeting, or maybe write letters for them. It makes it more difficult to offer a straightforward, therapeutic relationship. I've had this discussion with counsellors and at first, well, I thought they were being a bit precious, but I did a certificate myself in counselling and, yeah, now I can see that it isn't so much being precious, it's about creating and preserving that therapeutic relationship, that space for the client to simply be, and where the counsellor isn't, I don't know, stuck with other agendas, you know? So much mental health work is about monitoring and managing, and I know that's only part of it, of course we also work therapeutically, but the different roles mean it is hard to really get that purely therapeutic relationship.'

'So it feels to you as though the counsellor has a role in mental health, and you experience the effect of having a kind of multi-role responsibility, if that is what you mean?'

'Yes, it's the key working function which then merges with the treatment function and, as I say, the managing and monitoring, and liaison as well. As a key worker I may well be liaising with other agencies like social services, as well as with the psychiatrist. And so I am lots of different things to my client. And maybe what is helpful for some clients is to have someone who is simply their therapist, their counsellor, and maybe someone that they can actually talk to about frustrations over their treatment, just to be able to say it and be heard without feeling it will be passed on, you know?'

Alec nodded, aware that the topic of conversation – if it was right to describe a counselling exchange as a 'conversation' – was now much more of a 'co-professional' discussion or exploration. Yet he felt that perhaps this was OK. In a way it was a bit like what Merle had just said – clients needed a place to talk about their treatment and maybe here was a place for Merle to talk about the issues she had with the treatment she offered, and with her role in general.

'Space to just say whatever they want on any subject, without concern that it will somehow get back and affect their treatment.'

'I just think that we still have a long way to go to working out how the medical and therapeutic models can complement each other. And some places have maybe got it working better than others. I feel we may be a little too proscriptive, a little too "manage and contain" in our emphasis, and yet we work with people who are at risk to themselves and some of whom – albeit a small minority – could be a risk to others.'

'There are a lot of issues, a lot of tensions and demands being placed on you. How do medical and therapeutic models complement each other, how do you manage and contain risky patients in a therapeutic way? Big and challenging questions.'

'And ones that I think need to be asked because I think our clients need more than is often offered, and so we end up managing risk more than the client. I mean, if we are not careful, treatment becomes "risk-centred" rather than "client-centred", and I know that what we call client-centred in the NHS others might regard as "treatment-centred".'

The focus on 'risk-management' is important. Risk managers have been appointed in NHS trusts and risk registers have been written to highlight, evaluate and monitor risk. But there is a danger that services become so 'risk-minded' that the ability to take risks gets stifled.

By this is not meant clearly dangerous and unprofessional acts, but a culture that constrains the practice of 'thinking and acting out of the box' can develop. It can deter spontaneity and, in areas of therapeutic work, this is often the factor that makes all the difference in a therapeutic relationship. It can be said, 'life is a risky business'. Healthcare is a risky business to be sure – you can get infected by MRSA when you enter hospital for a routine operation, or take drugs whose side-effects make you feel worse than the original problem, or worse, leave you addicted.

There needs to be a system for monitoring and minimising avoidable risk, but it can get to a point that it engenders fear for the possible consequences of taking risks.

Alec smiled. 'Well, yes, as a person- or client-centred therapist, I would have to hold my hand up on that one. I hear the phrase "client-centred" being used, but it isn't truly client-centred, and that saddens me because it weakens the meaning.'

'It's good to talk like this. It really is. Even in supervision it can be so treatment-orientated – who's doing what with whom, and why. There is very little time to explore things more philosophically. Maybe we need more of that. And time to bring more of our personal reactions in as well. We need a more holistic kind of supervision.'

'Supervision that's more personal as well as professional, and embracing time for philosophical exploration too?'

Merle nodded. Yes, she thought, that was what was missing. Supervision had become so clinical in the unit, and she knew that was important, of course. This was an important feature of Clinical Governance, but so were the other areas. They surely had value in the continuing professional development that was required, and for Merle it was clear that somewhere in that there was a need for continuing personal development as well.

The session continued with further discussion about Merle's role, what she found most challenging and most rewarding. She said a little about some of the patients she worked with and realised that the way Alec listened was enabling her to talk about them in a very different way to how she presented them in her group and one-to-one supervision, which was in a factual and structured way. She felt more relaxed, more able to speculate, not feeling or fearing she would be judged as having got something wrong or said the wrong thing. She left the session very thoughtful as to what her professional needs were. She wasn't sure what to do with this, but it had made a deep impression.

Alec was meanwhile sitting feeling that the therapy session had become a col-legial discussion and then moved into being a kind of supervision session. He wasn't sure whether that was OK, but it had happened, and, well, he was simply responding to what Merle wanted to bring to the session. It was, after all, NHS staff counselling and she was bringing work issues, well, her clients. He wondered how she had found his way of listening and responding? Perhaps she was checking something out for herself? Perhaps what she had found help-ful in therapy she wanted to check out in a kind of supervision focus. He didn't know, but he was prepared to accept that Merle needed to have been the way she was, and felt sure that she would bring back any questions to their final session the following week.

Supervision session 2: processing therapist incongruence

Alec had been discussing another of his clients with Bernadette. Interestingly a young man called Paul who had issues around his sexuality, and who was seeking to come to terms with who he was and what he wanted. The theme had emerged in supervision of how the client had felt he needed a counsellor who was gay, and had been put in touch with Alec because of this. Talking about this with Bernadette had reminded him of the discussion with Merle in their last session, and when he had finished exploring his developing counselling relationship with the young man he moved on to Merle.

'It's this issue of what is most helpful, and realising we just don't know, we just don't know. With Paul it does somehow seem clear that he wants a gay counsellor, he feels he needs his difficulties heard by a gay man. And with Merle, she felt at first she would have preferred a black, female counsellor, and got me! And is now glad that she did.'

'Well, for me it's about the person, and if the person is right, if they offer the right conditions, and bring a certain quality of heart into the therapeutic relationship, then growth happens. And yes, people have preferences and they should be respected where possible. In a way, that respect is a therapeutic response. Sometimes people don't get what they think they want, it's not always available, but where there is choice, where a client has options, then I think they should be free to make it.'

'Well, Merle seems pleased.'

'You've obviously done a good job. How is it for you?'

'It feels good. I have watched her grow, watched her find her voice, watched her take action against the oppression she is experiencing in her place of work.'

'Great. And how many sessions now?'

'Seven sessions attended, one cancellation, one final session to go. And it already feels as though we have moved out of a purely therapeutic relationship.'

'How do you mean?' Bernadette wanted to clarify exactly what Alec meant by that. Was he overstepping a professional boundary? Did he mean it had got personal in some way? That was a daft thing to think, all therapy is personal, but there was personal and there was personal.

'The last session we really got into a discussion about working with clients, how the medical and therapeutic models could complement each other, and it actually began to feel more like a supervision session, with Merle talking about her work with some of her clients!'

'It happens. How was that?'

'It seemed fine, felt like a natural moving-on in some way. She'd talked about the grievance meeting she'd had – I'd better bring you up-to-date. She decided to raise the matter with her line-manager, which she did.'

'Wasn't she really struggling to decide what to do?'

'Yes, she was. I wouldn't say she was ambivalent, the tension was too dynamic, but she was feeling so exhausted and overwhelmed by work that it took a week on holiday with a friend for her to get some energy and sort of step back from it all and get a clearer perspective.'

'So, she kind of got away and took a deep breath and . . . ?'

'and went to her manager. He wasn't as sympathetic as she had hoped so she put in a formal grievance and has now had a formal interview with the service manager.'

Bernadette nodded. 'She's really found her voice?'

'That's how it seems, and that's how she sees it. She had to work through some of the messages from her aunt about keeping quiet, accepting things, how did she put it, something about her doing the Lord's work, and that so long as she was doing that everything would be OK. Got us into some interesting stuff about attitudes, generational differences and her feeling that she had to make a stand, not just for herself, but for others.'

'Sounds like you've had some interesting sessions!'

'We have, and it's been difficult as well, and there are some issues I need to talk through. But first, the sort of supervision session that she had with me, it felt OK, it felt like she was maybe exploring a different way of talking about her clients, and I didn't check it out but let it run. Seemed to me it was what she wanted, maybe needed, and so I went with it. But I just wonder, was it appropriate? Should I have said that this feels like supervision, and I wonder how that is? Or maybe I need to say that next time.'

'Were you feeling that at the time?'

'Well, no, it felt right, I mean, I was aware of the shift, but I felt well, it is the NHS and maybe this is OK. It's what my client wants to use the time for. She's worked on the issues she brought and maybe this is good use of time. But I think I could have checked it out.'

'So, you think you could have checked it out, but didn't.'

'No.' Alec stopped and thought about it. A thought had come to mind. 'Maybe I didn't want to check it out. Maybe I wanted it to become a supervision session.' Somehow that felt a little uncomfortable to say, but it also felt like it was close to the truth.

'You wanted to offer a supervision session to Merle?'

'Maybe, maybe I wanted her to get an experience of person-centred supervision, you know?'

Bernadette smiled. 'The salesman in you, huh?'

Alec laughed, 'Yes, something like that. You know me, I do get passionate about the approach.'

'I think we all do, it just comes out in different ways. I guess what's important is that you are aware of this tendency and, well, the need to watch that you're not imposing it on your clients.'

'I don't think I did, I just didn't question or stop it, and I suppose the question for me is whether I should have done, professionally speaking. And in a sense I know that I should have so the question is why didn't I, and how do I make sure that on another occasion I do say something?'

'Do you often work with clinicians, or is it usually managers or administration people, or ancillary staff who come to counselling?'

The supervisor has not held Alec on his previous comment through an empathic response. She has asked a question directing him towards a specific focus. She has moved away from a person-centred style of supervision.

'A mix. You think I saw an opportunity to "sell" the person-centred approach?'

'Just a wonder.'

'Not consciously.'

'OK, but to do it unconsciously means there was a measure of incongruence for you, you were doing something, communicating something without being fully aware of, or in touch with, your process.'

'Hmm, that's not easy to hear. I like to think I'm congruent.'

'We all do, but the challenge of the approach is being open to admitting that we aren't always, and I'm not sure we can be, always. There are always areas of ourselves that remain unexplored, life's a journey, we gain new experiences, we grow, develop and yes, get adversely affected as well by experiences. So I hear you saying that it's difficult to hear that maybe some incongruence emerged, but let's be glad that it has been recognised and therefore as a result of being aware of it it can be a little more congruent.'

'I suppose so. I mean I know that it's something we have to keep working at, but I guess it's when something happens that you miss, makes you wonder what else you might be missing.'

'Show me a truly congruent counsellor? Really.' Bernadette had opened her eyes wide as she spoke. 'We do the best we can, we endeavour to be accurately aware of our experiencing and to communicate what is present for us when it is felt to be therapeutically appropriate. We do the best we can. Didn't Rogers say in that Dublin interview something about being fortunate when empathy and unconditional positive regard are present, or are experienced by the client, something like that.'

'Yes, I know, you're right. Yes, thanks for putting it in perspective. I have to watch myself, I am passionate about the approach, and I have to say that I hope the bit of supervision did make a positive impression.'

> The counsellor needs to focus on the work with their clients, not in trying to prove an approach is best. It can be tempting, particularly where a counsellor does have a passionate belief in an approach, but the best way of conveying its power and effectiveness is by doing the work. A good theoretical approach will 'sell itself', whatever the theory. Alec has an issue here that he needs to be aware of, and needs to ensure it does not affect his work with clients but he needs to be careful not to lose his passion for his work and his approach. As ever, it is a balancing act.

Alec nodded and continued. 'Yes, you're right. And the fact that it occurred towards the end of the sessions, and with the more pressing issues dealt with – I don't mean completely resolved, but perhaps enough for the client to no longer feel so uncomfortable with them – she's more accurately in touch now I think with what she feels, and has shifted her locus of evaluation towards a more internal focus as well. At least it hasn't cut across the therapeutic process although I guess it is part of the process.'

'Sure. OK, so, anything else? You said something about wanting to discuss other issues as well.'

'Yes. Two things, both of which left me cutting across the therapeutic process with my stuff, once unwittingly, and once with awareness.'

'Go on.' Bernadette settled herself in her chair, aware that she was intrigued as to what Alec had been up to.

'She talked about her aunt dying in hospital and it flipped me across to my memory of my grandfather, and I got lost in my own thoughts and then I ended up saying something about knowing what it was like to lose someone special, something like that, and the focus ended up on me, and it just cut across the flow. It left me feeling disconnected from my client, and she seemed to lose her way as well, and it was just totally inappropriate. It really was an example of my stuff getting in the way.'

'So you found yourself thinking about your grandfather, and did you voice this?'

'Merle asked me what I had been thinking about, I think that was what she said, or maybe I said something about losing someone special. I can't recall exactly, but it did disrupt the flow. We got back into it again, the focus went back to Merle and her aunt, but for a while we were all over the place, at least, that was how it felt.' Alec paused, he remembered something, 'yes, and Merle said something about feeling the psychiatric nurse in her wanting to respond to me, but she didn't want that, she didn't want that side of herself in the session, that it wasn't for that. No, she didn't say it quite like that, but it was that kind of thing.'

'So your loss drew out the nurse in her, but she didn't want that.'

'No. And she looked lost, confused. I really think she was focused in an area of herself and then suddenly, because of what happened to me, she was jolted into another part and it was disorientating to her, and I lost the connection.'

'And the focus was then recovered?'

'It was. But it shouldn't have happened.'

'No, but it can and does happen. Sometimes we are affected by something and we are into it before we have a chance to contain it. The problem may be around your decision to share your experience. Or maybe it was the way you said it and, of course, the way your client heard it.'

'Yes, I mean, I didn't have to disclose anything, I could have just said that she had triggered a memory and then I could have brought the focus straight back, and yet, I don't know, there was a sense that it was important to say what I said. I mean, Merle did say that it was good to hear something about me, that's right, but it was then she frowned and said about feeling the psychiatric nurse in her emerging which she didn't want.'

'So the difficulty was around the part of her that emerged in response to what happened, it was that sudden emergence that disorientated Merle, perhaps?'

'Maybe, I don't know. Maybe you're right. And maybe it made something clear to Merle because she would have been experiencing a contrast in herself, and noting what she didn't want to bring into the session. So maybe it had some value, but I don't want that to be a kind of justification. The reality is I drifted off, and I self-disclosed, and both could have been avoided.'

'Mhmm, that's how it feels, you could have avoided both.'

'I wonder if I have issues related to my grandfather I need to address, that's the first thing. He was someone I really did look up to, he seemed to be so patient, so, I don't know, I guess the kind of grandfather a boy would dream of having.'

'Really special, the kind of ideal grandfather for a boy to have.' Bernadette had decided to stay empathically in touch with Alec to enable him to explore his feelings and memories for his grandfather. Although she didn't want to turn the session into therapy, she well recognised that a certain therapeutic content was an important part of supervision, and the material being explored had specific relevance to the supervision work that was being reviewed.

There are times when it is quite appropriate for supervision to include a therapeutic focus like this. It is relevant to the client work being discussed, and is alive within the supervision session. Of course, if it dominates the session, or seems to be in need of more focus and exploration, than taking it to therapy is likely to be more appropriate, or an extra supervision session needs to be arranged to focus specifically on the issue.

Alec nodded. He was back in his grandfather's shed, and it was one of the boats that he had made that came to mind. It was green – why he had painted it that colour he did not know, but he could remember it clearly. It wasn't one of the models he still had, and it was the one that he regretted most not having, but it had been passed on to his brother and, well, his brother had broken it somehow. He remembered being so upset and angry when he had found out. He could still feel emotions now.

'I still have some pretty powerful feelings about him and, well, just thinking about a boat he made for me that my brother later broke. I still have feelings after all these years.'

'Meant a lot to you.'

Alec nodded again, thoughtfully. 'I have to be aware of that, and I think I need to address that elsewhere. It's clearly a sensitive place for me so I should be pleased I have been made aware of it.'

'Something of a gift, perhaps, from Merle? I was going to ask what you felt you had received from the work with her.'

'Maybe, but I think as well it has really been good for me to be affected by her issues, and for it to lead me to think about my own attitudes, and diversity issues. Our last "supervision" session was really good for that. And I think seeing her grow, change, find her own power and use it to make a difference has helped strengthen my faith in time limited working. And as well this idea that it is the relationship that is key, the actual offering of the conditions for therapeutic growth or constructive personality change, however we choose to describe it.'

Alec nodded. The supervision session moved on. Alec felt easier at having explored these issues with Bernadette and he remained aware that he needed to self-monitor and explore a little more in therapy his relationship with his grandfather.

Points for discussion

- How effective was Alec's application of the person-centred approach in session 8?
- Was the more co-professional, conversational tone of session 8 appropriate? Make the case for your conclusion.
- What are your thoughts on the significance of diversity in the counselling relationship?
- Did Alec make the best use of the supervision time? Do you feel that the topics covered where fully addressed? What more would you have wanted from the supervision had you been Alec?
- Write notes for both sessions.

CHAPTER 8

Counselling session 9: endings and preparation for new beginnings

Merle sat in the waiting room, very conscious that this was her last session. In a way she felt sad, it had been such an important experience for her, and yet she also felt that it was right to end now, that she had achieved what she needed to and, yes, she probably would think about another counsellor at some point, but for now she felt she had a lot to think about and she wanted to get on with her life with the thoughts and feelings that had emerged and developed as a result of the last few weeks.

Although the previous supervision session in a way hadn't really reached any specific conclusion on the issues discussed, it had left Alec feeling somehow clearer in himself, and more aware of what was present for him.

When he came out Merle stood up and followed him to the counselling room. Last time, she thought, it was very present for her as she sat down in the chair, back to the door, as she had done each week.

'So, final session. Anything in particular you want to focus on?' Alec felt they probably would have a period of wind-down and reflection, but he wasn't going to introduce that. He felt sure Merle would ask for what she felt she needed.

'I'm just aware that it is the last session. I'm really glad I came for counselling. So much has changed. I'd like to bring you up-to-date with what's happening at work and, well, maybe think a bit about "what next?".'

'OK, so, where do you want to begin?'

'Well, I think that words have been said to the team manager. He seems to have been very quiet this last week, and it's not just me that has noticed. He just seems to be, I don't know, less of an issue. I mean, he's around, but he's sort of less in your face, well, less in my face. No, generally, I think they've clipped his wings a bit. Whether it sticks, well, time will tell, of course.'

'So, he's more withdrawn and it feels like he's had his wings clipped, and the question of "will it last?".' Alec sought to maintain the focus on what Merle had been saying.

'Yes, and I feel, well, relieved I guess. I mean, it's still hectic and demanding, but, well, I'm really making the effort to take breaks and give myself time. It's not easy, I still get caught up in the "oh, I'll just do one more thing" attitude, and then time I had planned to use for some reflection, or a break outside gets lost again. But I am better than I was.'

'So, still as busy as ever but at times you are managing to make time for yourself, and at other times you don't.'

'But it's still so different to how it was, I mean, I'm different. And I am having lunch breaks. And I am going out. And I'm also making the effort to eat more healthily. There's a new organic place opened up and I've been there twice this past week, and plan to try and keep that up. I've also decided to go to the gym, and I get membership at a reduced rate through an Improving Working Lives initiative – I've started to look into that. So it's like these sessions have triggered me into making other choices.'

'Sounds like you are making some health choices now?'

Merle nodded. 'I think before I was simply doing what I had to do to survive. That was it. I couldn't see beyond that, and I was running myself down.'

'Mhmm, unable to see beyond the treadmill as it were.'

'Yeah, and you know, it's strange, but I talked about respect before, you know, about getting respect and not feeling respected or valued, and you know, I've realised that part of my problem and a really big part – was that I wasn't really respecting myself. I mean I did, but I didn't. Like I wasn't making healthy choices for me. I wasn't acting in ways that respected my health, my wellness.'

Alec nodded and smiled as he heard the word 'wellness'. Not a word often used, and it took him back to a guy he'd met some years before, Patch Adams, a US medical doctor and professional clown, who spoke about this concept of wellness, and who had written a book about an Institute[1] he had established with this idea at its heart. He put the thought aside, though made a mental note to look through that book again when he got a chance.

'Mhmm, not respecting yourself, your health, your wellness.'

'And I can't be like that, not any more. I mean, I can't. Life's too short. I can make other choices, even when I feel trapped, well, I can choose to get out, you know?'

'Mhmm, you can make choices to break free.'

'Yeah, I like my work, I really do, but it is tough, it is demanding, and, well, maybe it could be organised better. And there are resourcing problems. And there is a problem with the throughput of clients. And maybe that's how it is. I don't know if it is the same everywhere. Maybe. Maybe there are more resources in other places, I don't know. And maybe I'll change direction, do something different, still in mental health, but in another area. I've been thinking about that as well. I've said my piece where I am, but do I want to stay there? Do I see myself there forever – no, no, I don't. I'll do different things, I am sure, and maybe I need to be a bit freer in my thinking, you know?'

'Free your thinking, expand your horizons, do you mean?'

---

[1] Gesundheit! Institute, P.O. Box 3134, Hagerstown, MD 21741–3134, USA.

Merle nodded. 'I like children, and I get on well with young people. Maybe I should think about that. There's a lot of money coming into early intervention services for young people with what they call first-episode psychosis. Maybe I could look into that. And there's substance misuse. I mean, I already see clients who have alcohol problems and some who use, or have used, drugs, which has affected their mental health.' Merle paused. 'I'm saying that, but I'm also complaining about how demanding it is, and, well, maybe substance misuse is more demanding, I don't know.' Merle stopped speaking, aware that she was feeling quite animated.

Alec had noticed that Merle's voice had risen a little, there seemed to be enthusiasm in the midst of a certain level of uncertainty as she ranged across the different possibilities. He tried to capture it in his response.

'So many possibilities, lots to feel enthusiastic about even though I sense there is uncertainty as to what to do.'

'And you know, it doesn't matter, I guess I have time to do them all? That's the weird thing. I don't know, something has changed, shifted in me. Something is telling me that I don't have to put up with the same old shit.' She smiled. 'Hell, there's new shit out there to try and to experience as well!'

Alec smiled. 'Lots of it!' They both smiled.

Humour has a place in therapy. Laughter and smiles bring a sense of well-being. Laughing with a client can be as therapeutically valuable as crying with a client. It affirms the presence of an area of the client's experiencing, validates it. Laughter can have a liberating quality, a moment when concerns may be thrown off, albeit temporarily. An opportunity in which a client may momentarily experience what it is like to be free. It can sow a very important seed in the heart and mind of a client, particularly if their mood is such that they have not laughed or genuinely smiled for a long time. Obviously, counsellors don't make jokes of things all the time, but genuine, spontaneous humour arising within a session is a positive, self-affirming experience and can have enormous therapeutic value.

'But you know what I mean?'

Alec nodded, 'Yes, you've got a profession and it gives you possibilities to try new things, develop new skills, work in different environments with new colleagues and clients.'

'And I've always known that, I guess, but I guess I've felt so ground down of late that I lost sight of it. Now I've regained it, but it's different as well.'

'You've regained something but it feels different.'

'And it feels good.'

'It definitely feels good.'

The session continued with further exploration of the possibilities for Merle's future career. Time passed quite quickly and there was soon only five minutes left.

'So, you have some idea for the future, seems like you have a renewed energy.' Alec was responding to the general theme and tone of their dialogue over the last few minutes.

'Very much so, and I want to thank you again.'

'I appreciate that and I want to say as well that you have done the work, you have made the changes, you have acted on the thoughts and feelings that have emerged and clarified for you.'

'I guess so. And I guess, well, it's strange really, I mean, in a way I feel more motivated, and yet at the same time I don't feel so committed to my present role somehow. It's like, yeah, I'll do what I do, and I'll do it well, but I can see further ahead now. I'd lost that, like I was saying, I was surviving and that's not healthy for me. And I wonder how many others are experiencing that, not just in the NHS, but in other jobs, you know?'

Alec nodded. 'Maybe lots of people.'

'And people need this kind of experience, time to talk it over, to really get in touch with what they want and to feel encouraged to make it happen.'

'Was that how it felt for you, like you were encouraged in some way to take the actions that you have?'

Merle thought about it. Her instinct was to say yes, but she'd never actually been told to do this or do that. So was she encouraged? 'I don't know. I mean, yes, I have been encouraged, but not directly or specifically. It's like, yeah, it became what I needed to do, albeit at first somewhat uncertainly. I mean, I didn't know what I wanted to begin with, other than to stop feeling what I was feeling and for it all to be different, but that seemed so impossible that I guess I got lost in feeling flattened by it all, and exhausted by the constant struggle to keep going.'

'Sometimes we don't realise how exhausted, how flattened we have become, we sort of adjust or adapt to it and it becomes how it is. And we just keep going, that is until the day comes when we can't keep going any longer.'

'And then we crumple. I hadn't quite got there, but I was heading there, I can see that now. Maybe a few more weeks and months and, who knows?'

Alec nodded, 'feels like that was where you were heading.'

'So, yes, so much has changed. I just hope things stay easier at work, you know. And it was good to have felt listened to, heard, taken seriously. And thank you for being part of that.'

'I'm glad that things have changed for you, I really am, and I hope that you'll go forward from this experience, and, well, I hope that things work out well.'

'I hope so too. Thanks.' Merle paused having noticed the time. 'Well, nearly time for me to head off. Thanks again, Alec, it's been really helpful and I think you've also helped me think differently about counselling now that I have had this experience. I mean, you know, I can see what it is about.'

'Well, it's not for everyone, perhaps, but it can help, give people time, space, someone to listen to them, take them seriously, help them to become what they want to become.'

Merle was getting up. 'Thanks again, anyway.' She held out her hand and Alec responded.

'Take care of yourself and have a good life.'

'You too.' She turned and left, feeling a little choked as she headed along the corridor. Silly fool, she thought to herself, but she did feel the emotion, she was
sad. It had been an important time for her and now, now she had to keep
taking the steps she wanted to take. 'Have a good life.' Well, she'd certainly
try. Time for a short coffee break and then back into the fray, a new client
she'd seen for the first time the previous week for assessment, history of self-
harming, messed up by abuse in childhood, disordered personality, history of
not complying with treatment. Maybe he never got the treatment he needed.
Another messed up life in the day of a psychiatric nurse.

Alec sat at home that evening. He'd looked up the book that had come into his
mind during that last session. 'Wellness', that was the concept he wanted to
remind himself about. He was thumbing though the book, and read, 'wellness
is the sum of everything that makes us healthier. In the wellness model,
patients become responsible for their own health. The healthcare professional's
role shifts from that of mechanic fixing a breakdown to a gardener nurturing
growth, because wellness results from active participation that only the self
can give' (Adams, 1993, p. 108). Yes, he thought, and what contributes to
wellness? He read on: 'nutrition, exercise, wonder and curiosity, love (given
and received), creativity, giving some form of service'. He looked up from the
page, how do we get the concept of wellness into the mindset of a health service that is so disease-centred in so many ways? His eyes went back to the page.
'Wellness is not a fad. It is life insurance in the truest sense of the word. To live a
healthy life means living at maximum potential in order to benefit oneself and
one's work, family, and society. Health is the greatest of all assets, but it cannot
be purchased or hoarded. Wellness is a process, a journey during which we
choose which paths to follow. We cannot depend on health gained in the past;
it must be renewed each day' (Adams, 1993, p. 113).

Alec smiled as a thought crossed his mind. Wellness as a process, a journey.
Maybe that's how he should think of the actualising tendency, as a process, a
movement, an urging towards wellness. Rogers wrote of full functionality.
Maybe wellness is the process that can get us there.

Reflections

Merle's reflections – 'I was in such a different place when I started to come to the
counselling sessions. Thank goodness it was there. I don't suppose I would
have seen someone privately, not then. I would now, but I'm not the same
person. I seem to have woken up from a nightmare that I had drifted into without realising that it had happened. Now I can see things more clearly, or so it
seems to me.

'It was good to talk and to be listened to, really listened to. Yes, that made a deep
impression. Certainly made me think about my own work. How many of my clients tell me they don't feel understood, don't feel anyone gives them enough

time? Well, I can appreciate that in a more immediate way now. Being listened to, being heard, and being taken seriously, yes, that was really important.

'So now I am more settled in my job, things have remained better, and yet at the same time I feel more unsettled as well. Strange. But I know my time at the unit is limited. I will move on, not sure what to just yet, but I am keeping an eye on the adverts in the journals and the national press.

'So, what was the most significant part of the counselling? Not being told what to do was important, though at the time I wasn't really thinking about it. But I really did find my own way. I didn't feel any pressure. Even when I changed my mind and felt unable to confront the oppression in the NHS; my need to feel that way was accepted. No attempt was made to encourage me to feel differently. That was something that encouraged me and maybe it was more real for me.

'It's strange but I thought I'd have a lot to say. I usually do, but somehow there isn't much more to say. I feel different, I am different: more confident and more self-assured. I needed that time out and I think that maybe counselling should be more widely available in the NHS. It does promote healthier lives. It shouldn't be seen as something you go to as a last resort when everything has fallen apart. There needs to be a culture of, perhaps, regular time out to talk things over. I guess not everyone needs a counsellor for this; family and friends can provide it as well. But it isn't always appropriate, sometimes it is good to spend that time with someone you do not know, who has no agenda, and who can just let you range over all that's most pressing.

'So that's me, determined to continue taking coffee and lunch breaks, and to make choices in my life that make me feel well. I've also decided to move and share a flat with a couple of friends. That won't be easy, but I know I have to do it. Life at home is too unhealthy. I love mum, and I'll be there for her, but I have to be in a new environment where I feel I can grow. I was heading where she is, coping with life by retreating under the duvet cover. I have to be different. I have to make fresh choices, new starts. And my aunt? The tears are welling up in my eyes as I think of her. What would she think? I think she'd be proud of me, and would probably say that "all would be well".'

Alec's reflections – 'They were quite intense sessions. Gave me a lot to think about. Forced me to think about my own attitudes and the nature of inter-cultural counselling relationships. But I enjoyed them. It was good to see the changes occurring for Merle, and to hear that things were working out a little better at work. Whether it has stayed that way, I don't know.

'I look back over the sessions now and, yes, I made mistakes, I know I did. My stuff did get into the process – it happens. But sometimes it can be avoided and I think I have learned once again to be attentive to reactions within myself.

'I felt warmth for Merle, genuinely so. She really did look so low at times, so flattened by all that had happened. The one time you need the person you normally turn to and she's no longer there. But she found a way through. I like to believe that the therapeutic relationship created the experiential climate that allowed the shifts to occur. They have to come from within. I could have told her what to do, as could someone else, but it would not have been the same. Ownership is crucial, having the time to actually connect with the feelings and thoughts that are struggling to emerge but are buried under the concrete of oppressive attitudes.

'As a white man I am left with lots of feelings and thoughts around these issues. The white races have so much to answer for. I don't take it personally as I once did. But I do accept that I have responsibility to ensure, to the best of my ability, that I do not encourage oppressive or racist attitudes where I have influence.

'Working as a counsellor in the NHS brings me into contact with some wonderful people, really dedicated people who simply want to care, want to make that difference in the lives of people who are sick and unwell. The dedication is truly enormous. But it can be exploited and that isn't good. It leaves staff members torn. Where people are giving from the heart – and I have to say that I sincerely believe that the heart is an important factor in any healing process – then they are open to being affected by what is going on around them. People in caring professions are there because they care, because they carry a quality of heart that means they want to help. Of course, there are going to be those who are career clinicians and simply see it as a job, well, it's not for me to comment.

'So I am hopeful that Merle will now make a new start in her life, and maybe she will also be open to new possibilities. The counselling process we shared wasn't perfect, but it was as it was. I don't feel damage was done, far from it. But there's no reason to be complacent. As a person-centred counsellor I have to have a certain discipline and achieve that particular blend of the personal and the professional to be effective. I feel good about the process. And, yes, I feel passionate about the approach. I do believe that effective counselling is linked to the quality of the counselling relationship, and that, in turn, is linked to the heartfelt attitude of the counsellor.'

PART 2

The manager under stress

CHAPTER 9

Counselling session 1: a client overwhelmed and desperate for control

Gerald was looking at his watch as he hurried along the corridor. Late again. He thought he had time to check his email one last time for the day – he knew he wouldn't be heading back after the counselling session. But he hadn't expected the request for information that he had to attend to. Email, everything, seemed to be expected immediately. So as a result he couldn't get away as he had planned, and then the ward manager caught him on the way out. It never ended.

He'd already had the best part of a week off work, he had found it hard to cope and his manager had told him to go home and rest up. It had been a difficult few months – well, it seemed as though it had been difficult for Gerald, so much change, targets, resourcing problems, new staff, difficult staff and now Agenda for Change! What a name. Who needed an agenda for change, the NHS was in constant change. So, he'd rested up for the week, got out into the sunshine, tried to unwind, but here he was, back at work and after only two days caught up in the old problem of too much to do and not enough time.

He'd agreed to take up counselling. He wasn't sure whether he had the time, and that was the irony, of course, not having the time to take the time out to sort himself out. Anyway, he was nearly there now, only a few minutes late after all, but he was breathless.

He let the receptionist know that he had arrived and was directed into the waiting area. He sat down and caught his breath.

He had also been to see his doctor as well whilst he had been off the previous week. Turned out that his blood pressure was up and the doctor did one or two other tests and took some blood. Stress was the diagnosis. He would have referred him to the surgery counsellor but by then Gerald had already made contact with the service at the hospital. He'd sent staff there himself in the past, or at least encouraged them to go. They only accepted self-referrals. And he understood that they were good, so he wasn't concerned. But he hadn't been to counselling before and, well, he did have some anxieties, wondering quite what they would expect him to talk about. He did have a brief conversation with the counsellor that he would be seeing and he was grateful that there hadn't been a wait. He was surprised. He'd expected to wait. You waited for everything else these days. Though he understood he was lucky. There had been a cancellation. He was going to have an initial session and then be offered further sessions in a few weeks, that was the best they could offer. He'd accepted that, felt he needed to see someone straightaway, maybe start to sort things out rather than wait and then, well, he didn't want to end up having to take more time off.

A late middle-aged lady came into the waiting area. 'Gerald Andrews?'

Gerald looked up, 'yes, that's me.'

'Hello, I'm Barbara, we spoke on the phone.'

'Yes, yes we did.' He shook her hand.

'Won't you come through to the counselling room.'

'Thank you.' He followed her in and sat down.

'Sorry I'm a bit late, work, as ever.'

'Sure, no problem. I gather it's very busy.'

'It's always very busy, that's the problem.' Gerald smiled, although it was through slightly gritted teeth.

'So, when we spoke on the phone, I explained briefly about confidentiality, that unless you disclosed something that was clearly putting patients or anyone else at specific risk, everything would remain confidential to me, and between me and my supervisor.'

Gerald nodded. He understood, and he knew he had nothing he planned to say that would be likely to leave anyone needing to pass anything on. 'Yes, I appreciate that.'

'And today will be an initial session really, and then the next time I can see you is in three weeks. It's not ideal, but you said you'd prefer to start now and have a gap.'

'Yes, it actually suits me. I have a week's annual leave coming up so I'd have missed a week anyway.'

'OK. And that we have a maximum of six sessions.'

'Including this one?'

'Yes.'

'OK.'

'And the sessions are fifty minutes. We have about forty minutes left for today. How do you want to use the time?'

Gerald nodded. 'OK, well, where to begin.' He smiled.

'Not always easy to know.'

'No, I suppose I should say something about my work.'

'Mhmm.'

The person-centred counsellor will want the client to choose their focus and establish their own direction in the session. Having discussed confidentiality issues over the phone, it helps to leave the first face-to-face contact free for the client to focus. The client wants to talk about his work, so that is what

> the focus becomes. The counsellor trusts implicitly that the client knows what is most pressing for him. Other factors may emerge – they probably will. But it is not for a person-centred counsellor to start asking questions in order to elicit information that, quite simply, may not be what the client wishes to bring, at least, not at that time anyway.

'I'm a service manager in the hospital, responsible for overseeing the running of the Accident and Emergency Department, and I also have responsibilities for some areas of liaison, for instance with ambulance crews. I'm also covering for the orthopaedic ward as well at the moment. We have a staff vacancy that has not been filled and so some managerial roles have been distributed across different service managers. It hasn't helped.'

'So, a busy role and extra responsibilities as well.'

Gerald nodded. 'And, well, I don't know what happened but, well, I suppose it just got too much.' Gerald was staring ahead of him, feeling a little bit fuzzy in his thinking. He had so many things to think about that it was hard to really focus away from it.

'So, feeling overwhelmed by it all.'

'And, well, a couple of weeks back it got really crazy, we just had a particularly bad weekend. It was hot and, well, there must have been some frayed tempers. We had so many people coming through in the evenings, many were alcohol-related injuries, people fighting, falling over, passing out. I don't work evenings, but I get the paperwork across my desk, and the nurses in charge during the shifts reporting to me for the managerial aspects of their work. There had been an incident, an SUI: serious untoward incident – you know what I mean?'

Barbara nodded, 'yes'.

'Well, a fight had broken out in the Accident and Emergency Suite. A patient, drunk, had kicked off, and taken a swing at one of the junior doctors. It seems that in the confusion the patient got pinned down by a number of members of staff and the police were called, and it would appear that the patient sustained two broken ribs. At least, that is what he is alleging. Of course, when the incident occurred he hadn't been assessed, in fact he was coming through to be assessed by a duty doctor. So, I came in on Monday with all the allegations and counter-allegations, staff wanting to know what we were going to do about it – yet another incident, and wasn't there supposed to be "zero tolerance" of violence towards staff, so why did we let the drunks in? It seems as though it was a kind of final straw. I had to start writing a report and got so far with it and, well, I don't know, I just felt as though I'd lost it. I couldn't concentrate, found myself not wanting to deal with it, not wanting to know about it really. I had two sleepless nights and saw my manager on the Wednesday and he told me to take a break, he said I looked really grey and tired and I needed time to get myself back on track.' Gerald paused, being very aware of how he had felt. He had been so tired that day, and so anxious. 'I knew he was right but I didn't want to accept it, but he insisted, said he had a duty of care towards his staff and that I needed to look after myself. He'd sort out what needed to be done.'

Barbara had been listening attentively. She hadn't responded to anything that Gerald had been saying, in truth he hadn't really given her much of a chance. Everything just came out and it felt to her like a wave; the kind of wave that you get when there's a flood and it just sweeps through carrying everything with it.

'So, the incident, the report, the way staff were reacting.'

'I lost it. I know I did. I just couldn't stop thinking about it, worrying about it. I mean, it's not something I haven't dealt with in the past. These incidents happen and you produce an initial report of the incident that goes to the risk management department and a decision is taken as to whether it will then be investigated further, which, of course, it would be given the nature of what happened. Fine, so you set the process in motion, interview staff, get statements, pull it all together, establish what happened and what could be learned from it and make recommendations which then feed into an action plan. But staff were sounding off and, well, I don't know, I lost it and somehow it just got to me, not just that, just the whole everything about the department.' He sighed and shook his head. 'So here I am. I had the rest of the week off and the weekend and now I'm back but already I can feel it again. The doctor wanted to sign me off for a couple of weeks when I saw him, but I said no, I'd be OK, I'd take it easy. He told me my blood pressure was up and that I was displaying symptoms of stress. So ... the report is still in process though my manager has said that he will continue with it. And I need to try and make sure it doesn't all get on top of me again. I'm seeing him again tomorrow and I hoped for some ideas from today.'

Barbara nodded. 'So much going on, so much to deal with. Under stress and hoping for some ideas to, what, make your work more manageable?'

'Yes, I suppose so, although I know what you do to avoid stress, you know, organising your day, having breaks, making sure you get out of the building at lunch-time, exercise, diversionary interests, supervision, prioritising work, all that, but, well, I've sort of stopped doing it I guess. I seem to spend the day rushing from one thing to the next. I just never seem to be able to stop.'

'So these kinds of things you had in place but now they've got lost somewhere.'

'Yes, yes they have. I don't have the time, and that's crazy, but I don't. And I find it hard to switch off at home. My wife tells me I'm unbearable in the evenings. I can't sleep. A large scotch used to help, but now that doesn't seem to work any more.'

By maintaining simple, straightforward empathy, the client has been able to flow with his stream of thinking, and it has taken him through work and into his home life. This is a more natural flow of disclosure than a question and answer session. The client will feel in control, he is setting the scene, he is deciding what he wants to disclose and when. He is being listened to and hopefully he is experiencing this.

His alcohol use has also been disclosed, easily, without pressure. The client does not see it as a problem and not a great issue is made of it, the counsellor later making a comment, flagging up an issue related to it. Alcohol use is a common response in dealing with stress. Yes, it relaxes, but its mood altering affect comes with a cost – over time more is needed for the same affect, and its addictive nature begins to assert itself. Organisations need clear alcohol (and drug use) policies and counselling and human resources staff need skills and knowledge in working in this area.

'So you drink scotch in the evening to help you sleep in the past, and still do, but it doesn't help any more?'

'No, it doesn't.'

Barbara thought to herself that, well, she quite appreciated that that could happen if one drank quite a lot on a regular basis. The temptation would be to drink more to chase the effect. 'Alcohol can help you sleep, but it can disturb sleep patterns as well.'

'Well mine are all over the place.'

'So, your sleeping is affected and that leaves you tired during the day, and things are difficult at home because of how you are.'

'So my wife says. I just want time to unwind. But there's always some noise in the house. The kids are around – they're both teenagers – God help us. Music, phones going, televisions on, the doorbell as friends come round. It never stops. I actually delay going home now, stop off at the pub for a couple of pints.'

'So you've found a way of giving yourself a bit of a break, bit of a transition between work and home.'

Gerald nodded. 'But it's not good. I'm getting later and later, the wife's having a go, we're not really communicating much these days. I don't know, it's all too much. I just can't seem to get a grip on myself, or on anything for that matter.'

Barbara felt herself wondering what it must be like for his wife as well. Both of them under stress. The relationship under stress. She kept her empathic response focused on what Gerald had been saying. 'So you stay longer in the pub, your wife has a go at you about it, communication feels as though it is breaking down and everything just seems to be, I don't know, you can't seem to get a grip of it.'

'I can't, and that's not me. I'm organised, I know how to be organised, I know how to organise my day. I'm a structured person, but I can't seem to, I don't know ... I just don't know.' He sat back in the chair, slumped would be a more accurate term, as if he had exhausted himself of all he had to say.

Barbara allowed all that had been said to make its impression upon her, whilst she also acknowledged her own reactions as well. Something has to change here, she thought to herself, or else someone is going to end up very unwell and the marriage is going to be under real threat. But it wasn't her role as a person-centred counsellor to start making assumptions and seeking to address them. She accepted that Gerald was doing what he needed to do to hold himself together. She voiced her thoughts. 'You're doing what you need to do to keep yourself together but it feels like it just isn't working, and it's getting more and more out of control.'

'I know.' He stared blankly ahead of him, his head bursting.

'So you want to regain that control but you just don't know how to at the moment?' Barbara asked the question tentatively.

> The counsellor has introduced the word 'control'. She does so tentatively. She has allowed all that has been said by her client to make an impression. Her response is not hurried, but a paced expression of what she genuinely feels, senses, experiences as a result of listening to her client. It proves to be a significant word, facilitating the client to powerfully connect with his feelings about control and lack of it.

'I have to be in control.' He stared at Barbara, shaking his head slightly from side-to-side, it was a kind of tension movement, a sort of despairing shake. 'I have to, I have to . . .'

'You have to regain control, you have to.' Barbara kept her response simple. She was not there to problem-solve, but to ensure that what Gerald talked about was heard and accepted, and that he was enabled to engage with his thoughts and feelings as fully as he found possible. She knew he would have the answer, but it was buried, hidden, lost under the stress reactions, the anxiety, the sleeplessness, the almost traumatised effect of being in a situation where you felt you were no longer in control – of what was going on around you and of your own reactions.

Gerald felt so desperate to have control. His life felt like it was running away from him, a runaway train and he didn't know whether to get on or jump off. He wanted things to be better at home, he loved Maggie, his wife, and their two children – John and Michelle – but he was losing them and he didn't know what to do . . .

He felt the strength of the emotion, the pain and despair, and he fought back the tears. He wasn't going to cry, he had to keep in control, it was the only way, the only possible way to come through this.

'I shouldn't be like this. I know work is demanding.' He used work to push aside his feelings for his family. This was counselling in the context of his work, he felt he had to talk about work. No one had told him this, but it was what he felt he should do. 'And, OK, it is busy, busier than it has been, but I've always coped. I've never been like this before, ever.'

Barbara nodded, 'it's a new experience for you. Everything is OK, manageable, and then suddenly it isn't. You've always coped and then suddenly . . .' She left the sentence unfinished, feeling that she had conveyed her empathy and wanting to allow Gerald to remain focused on how it was for him, now, as he sat with her with all the overwhelming and stressful thoughts and feelings within him.

'So I don't know. I have to get a grip on it all, I have to. I just feel, I don't know, sometimes I . . .' Gerald's thoughts went from his desk and the piled up in-tray to members of staff who were under pressure, then to Maggie, John and Michelle. He felt sadness in his despair. The feelings were very present.

To Barbara it was clear that Gerald had a lot on his mind, and she felt his despera-
tion, of not knowing which way to turn. She knew that at this moment he was
very much in the awfulness of his experience, maybe connecting more strongly
with his feelings. She knew that until he truly owned what he felt it was unlikely that he would truly move on, at least, that was how she saw it. So many
problems are because people are not allowing themselves to feel what is present
within them. People push feelings aside, reasonably so because they feel too
overwhelming to get close to, and once they start pushing one set away then
others can become more remote as well.

'. . . sometimes you?'

'Just want to walk away from it all, just take off, leave it *all* behind.'

'Leave it *all* behind?' Barbara matched Gerald's emphasis.

'No, not everything, but work, yes, work. I'd like to just walk out of the office
one day and say, "that's it, I've had enough, I'm going to do what *I* want to
do now".'

'That's powerful, to say you've had enough and you want to do what *you* want
to do.'

'Yes, but it doesn't work like that, does it?'

'That how it feels, doesn't work like that?'

'No, but it feels good thinking about it.'

'Mhmm. Good to think about the idea of walking out and doing something different, something for you.'

The client connects with important and satisfying thoughts and feelings.
Yes, he would like to walk away and do something different. He may, or
may not, have an idea what that something is, but he is allowing a part
of his experience to be present in his awareness, and is communicating it to
the counsellor. He is in a state of congruence with respect to the idea of
moving on.

It has to be remembered that whilst congruence is sometimes thought of
as referring to the whole person, his or her whole experience being accurately present in awareness, the reality is that it is usually more about specific experiences. He may or may not act on what he is aware of experiencing
in himself, that is the next step, the next decision, but what person-centred
counselling encourages is for clients to be more fully and accurately aware
of themselves, of their experiences as a person, from which they can then
make more informed choices rooted in authenticity, in what *they* think and
feel based on *their* evaluation of circumstances, factors and experiences.

'Not just for me, for Maggie as well, and the kids. Something different, get away
from the . . . , oh I don't know, I guess you can't. The kids are at school, they're
settled. Maggie's got her own work, it's me, I'm the one that wants something
to change.'

'So they're OK with how things are, do you mean, but you want change?'

'Well, no, I can't imagine they're happy. Maggie and I row, well, I guess that's normal, but it's tense. She doesn't understand the pressure I'm under.'

'So you think they probably aren't happy with the way things are.'

Gerald shook his head, 'no, no, I can't go on like this, it's got too much, I have to make some changes somehow.' He lapsed into silence, somehow a little clearer in his knowing that he needed to make changes, but at the same time still very much not knowing what changes to make.

'So, you have to make changes, alter things a bit.'

He wanted to change things at home. But he knew he needed to be different for that to happen, and the thing that made him how he had become was work. That was the problem. 'It's work, it just feels too much.'

'So, work is the root of the problem, the demands on you are too much.'

'I think it's been coming on for a while.' Gerald hadn't really thought about it quite like that before, but somehow that was how it felt, and that was how he heard himself describing it. 'I guess it's been building up but, well, you keep going, don't you?' He nodded his head and took a deep breath. 'I need to make some changes, and I need a longer chat with my manager as well. We have flexible working schemes and maybe I need to look at that, maybe there can be some flexibility somehow, I've got to break the pattern I've got stuck in.'

Barbara noted the change of tone, a sense of direction was emerging, a movement away from the 'I don't know' that had been very much a feature of the way Gerald had been speaking. She said, 'so look at ways of changing that pattern.'

'I need space, that's what I need, when I was saying about walking away from it all, or something like that, the image I had was of space, big areas of space, countryside stretching away before me and the sky above, blue sky, clear, sunshine on my face and a cool breeze.' He smiled. 'You don't see a lot of sunshine in A&E, and my journey to work isn't through the countryside. Wish it was. I've never been able to travel to work through countryside.'

'So something about open countryside and sunshine on your face.'

'And a cool breeze, you know, that's important.'

Barbara smiled. 'So, how do you feel now as you think about this?'

'A bit wobbly inside but, yes, it feels good.'

'Wobbly but good.'

'Yes, I can feel, oh it's hard to describe, but it's like a kind of trembling.' He could feel it. He lifted his right hand. It was trembling, he could feel it, see it. 'Look at that, see?' he shook his head. 'I need to relax, I really do. I'm not doing myself any good the way things are. I'm getting into habits that I can well do without.'

'Such as?'

'Going to the pub every evening. That really isn't helping. I mean, it helps to wind me down, but it makes things more difficult at home. No, I need to try and do something about that, but that means coping better with the stresses from work.'

In the space of a few minutes the client connects with powerful imagery for what makes him feel good, and then an area of particular concern emerges. He wants to travel to and from work in the countryside, in the sunshine, but he comes home via the pub. The counsellor lets him flow with it. He is experiencing contrasts in himself, which he must make his own judgements about. He doesn't have to actually then discuss the contrast, he has experienced it, he knows it. What will take shape as a result only time will tell. The person-centred counsellor knows she does not have to 'do' anything to make this process happen. As the client is offered the freedom to move around within himself, his own awareness is contrasting experiences. The person-centred counsellor accepts that this is a trustworthy process, flowing at its own pace, and which will induce the emergence of thoughts, feelings and actions when the time is right. The person-centred counsellor works with the client's process, with their timing, with, if you like, the inherent purposefulness to induce fuller functionality and greater satisfaction from the existence of the actualising tendency. Person-centred counselling creates the relational climate to stimulate this.

'Mhmm, so it comes back to work and the demands being placed on you.'

'And, I mean, I think the NHS is good at helping people. I've certainly had to work with staff on ways of dealing with workload – always seems easier to solve someone else's problems!'

'Mhmm. Harder when it comes to your own.'

'I'm going to talk to my manager again, see what we can work out. Maybe, I don't know, maybe a shorter working day might help, earlier start, earlier finish, I don't know, that doesn't really appeal either, or a late start, late finish.' He smiled to himself. 'I guess what I want is a late start and an early finish!'

'Has its appeal, but that feeling really says something about how work is affecting you.'

'Yes, I don't want to be there more than I have to be. Maybe I've been in the job too long. But it's only been a couple of years. But then, something new would have its stresses as well.'

'So a sense that a change of job, although it has some appeal, might not really resolve feeling stressed?'

'And I don't like the idea of being stressed, it feels like being weak. I mean, being stressed means you're not coping. OK, I know I'm not coping too well, but stress implies that you can't cope. I believe I can, it's getting through this and making changes.'

Barbara nodded and noticed that the session would soon have to end. She wanted to check whether it had been helpful.

'Time's coming up, so I wanted to check whether this has been helpful.'

Gerald nodded and replied, 'Yes, yes it has. Just being away and talking. I thought I might have more, I don't know, specific ideas, but then we haven't really got into specifics, and maybe that's something to discuss with my manager anyway. I'm glad you were able to fit me in, even though there is a break until the next one. I think it's been important to come, and, well, with a week's holiday coming up maybe that will give me more time to think and see how things are when I come next.'

'OK, so let's sort out the date and time of the next session.'

After Gerald had left, Barbara sat and pondered on the session. She felt tired, more so than usual. The session had felt intense. She didn't feel she had said a great deal, very much a case of not getting in her client's way, allowing the flow to continue as he needed it. She was pleased that he had come out of the session with a few positive thoughts, and that maybe he was a little clearer. It was always hard to be sure, but he had seemed OK with the session.

Once again she noted how work issues so often lead into issues outside of work. Clearly there were relationship problems at home, and how much that was related to how Gerald's work affected him, well, Gerald seemed to think that it was. She saw a lot of clients struggling with stress, this kind of overload. Often people ended up discussing things with occupational health, particularly when it reached the point that they were having to take time off. Maybe that would follow, she didn't know. At the moment she simply felt positive about the connection she had made with Gerald, and that in spite of feeling overwhelmed he had a certain intention to fight back. In that she admired his resilience whilst also noting to herself that often too much resilience meant that when someone finally did overload they came down heavily and could then take longer to recover.

She remembered reading something describing stress in terms of being like an electric circuit that you overload by plugging too many things in. You just keep adding more and more and eventually the trip switch is activated. You reset it, and pretty soon you have turned everything back on and it trips again. Until you start to reduce the amount turned on it will continue to trip. You either need to get the electrician to make changes to the wiring to cope with the extra load, or you have to find ways of managing with less on the circuit. She was never sure whether she was the electrician called in to try and change her patient's wiring, or the person called in to help someone decide what they could, or couldn't, switch on! She guessed she was a bit of both. Some clients wanting to make lifestyle changes to help them carry a greater load, others wanting to simply reduce the load.

Gerald, meanwhile, was heading back to work. He had felt a little more relaxed when he'd been talking about the countryside and having space, but as the session had drawn to a close, and now, he could feel his anxiety creeping up again. He knew he had to talk to his manager. Something had to change. At least he only had next week and then a week away. He needed it, the whole family needed it. They were heading over to France to stay with friends in a place they'd bought and renovated. Yes, it would be good to get away, and he was so glad that it was planned. He just had to get through the next ten days.

Supervision session 1: the significance of contact

'I have a new client. Not much to say at the moment. He's referred himself
   because of stress at work. Service manager in an Accident and Emergency
   Department at the hospital in town. What a job.'
Colin, her supervisor, could only imagine what it must be like to work in an envir-
   onment like that. He admired people who stuck at what he felt must be difficult
   jobs, glad that somebody did them, and also glad that it wasn't him.
'That must be a tough one.'
'Yes, and he has responsibilities for another ward because of staff shortages.'
Colin raised his eyebrow and took a deep breath. 'So, he's burned out, huh?'
'Heading that way if things don't change, I think. He's already had some time off.
   His manager told him to go home and rest up.'
'An enlightened manager.'
'I think, by the sound of it, he'd reached breaking point, and then there had been
   an incident and, well, it was too much.'
'Incident?'
'A drunk patient and, well, staff restrained him, and the patient is now alleging
   his ribs were broken during the restraint. So, well, incident report and a man-
   agement report required. That seemed to be the thing that did it.'
'So, he's still off?'
'No, back at work. I saw him quite quickly because there had been a cancellation,
   but he has to wait for three weeks for the next appointment.'
'Is he OK with that? Are you OK with that?'
'He has a week's holiday anyway coming up, so, yes, I think it's OK and he seems
   OK with it.'
'So, I have a sense of the issue though not all the specifics, but little sense of your
   client.'
'I guess that says something, doesn't it? The work stuff is more in the foreground.
   I guess that's how it is for Gerald – that's his name.'
'OK, so, yes, clearly it made an impression on you because it is what you have
   told me.'
'I feel like I'm passing it on.'
Colin was interested. These kinds of feelings could often say a lot about the issue
   that had arisen in the counselling sessions, and the way that the counsellor
   was handling it. 'So, you want to pass it on. Something about it that makes
   you want to do this?'

Often the way a counsellor experiences themselves as they discuss a client,
or reconnect with their experience of being with a client, can arouse sensations that can be valuable in understanding the therapeutic process
and relationship that is developing. Barbara's sense of wanting to pass
something on is explored, allowing her to become more aware of what is

> present for her, material that she might not otherwise have dwelt on and acknowledged. It is important, for the sake of preserving congruence, to have a clear awareness of what impact a client is having on the counsellor.

Barbara thought for a moment or two. 'It's not that it's hot, you know, or sharp, something that you grab hold of and immediately want to let go of. It's not like that.'

'So it's not like a sudden, intense experience.'

'No, it's more about heaviness, the weight of it all.' She paused. 'Or is it?'

'Something about heaviness and weight that doesn't sound quite right?'

'I was thinking that things can be small and heavy, but it doesn't feel small because it's affecting all areas of his life.'

'So it's as much about the size as the weight, is that what you mean?' Colin was checking out, seeking to clarify what Barbara was experiencing, though he immediately felt concern that he was perhaps putting words into her head when maybe she would be better finding her own.

'It's heavy, but more psychological than physical, and, no, not even something I'm holding, it's more like a really thick, heavy cloud, a fog, but there's weight there as well, a burden. So, yes, the image of walking in a fog somewhere with a weight on your back. And yes, and this is because of something Gerald talked about, but there are tall buildings, you feel hemmed in with it, trapped, unable to find a way out.'

'That's really impressive.'

'Once I start in on it, well, I guess I have an active imagination!'

'Well, maybe, but you've had, how many sessions with this client?'

'One.'

'And yet you can describe it with such powerful imagery.'

'So either I'm being overly imaginative or it really is something quite immense that has made an impression on me?'

'What do you think?'

'I don't know. I did feel drained after the session. I often do, but I particularly felt that way after seeing Gerald.'

'So it's really heavy stuff that Gerald is going through.'

'Yes, and not just at work, it's affecting his marriage and his home life, and he's got into the habit of dropping in at the pub after work to unwind, and that's upsetting his wife. And he's drinking more which is upsetting his sleep pattern. It's potentially a real mess.'

'And could get a lot worse.' Colin was thinking about how, in his experience, the kind of pattern that Barbara was describing could lead to really big problems, particularly once alcohol had become a coping mechanism. More stress, more alcohol, less quality sleep, lowering mood, reduced resilience to stress, more alcohol, and so it could go on. He'd listened to people telling him how they'd lost everything following that kind of path. At least Gerald seemed to be addressing it early. So often this kind of issue came to light when someone was found to be alcohol-affected at work, and then, rather than a supportive response, a disciplinary route would be followed. Oh well, that was his experience, he knew it wasn't always like that, but that it could be.

'I haven't responded to the alcohol side of it. He seems to have noted for himself that it is a problem.'

'Good. Like everything, we make choices to try and feel better, to try and maintain ourselves and our self-concept. That's what he's been doing, trying to keep himself going as a manager, but as a husband, well, that's maybe been pushed into second place. And I don't want to lose what you were saying about the heaviness and the cloud, and you mentioned buildings.'

'Gerald had said about how sometimes he wanted to walk away from it all. I clarified whether he meant all by empathising with his use of the word, and he said no, but he had this image of the countryside, of open space, sun on his face, and a cool breeze, he seemed to particularly note that.'

'Well we can speculate on that, though it will be our view, not his meaning, of course.'

'I see it as something refreshing. I guess it feels psychologically hot – not sure what I mean by that – given where Gerald works.'

'That would make sense. So, he has a clear image as well. Maybe imagery, and perhaps metaphor, may form a significant element in the counselling dialogue you will be having with Gerald.'

'I hadn't thought of it quite like that, but maybe, though I won't introduce it but maybe I'll be ready to accept that if it arises from Gerald – it may be particularly important to him.'

'So, what, the usual six sessions?'

Barbara nodded.

'Any issues with that?'

'No, I'm used to it. We'll see how it goes. I'm sure that a lot can be achieved; it's up to Gerald. At least, in spite of feeling overwhelmed, he seems motivated, he wants to make changes even though he's not sure exactly what.'

'That's positive. But, well, if he had needed to feel unmotivated then you would have needed to have respected that as well.'

'Quite, though that's where the NHS workplace agenda can make an impact.'

'Can you say more?'

'Well, NHS staff counselling is supposed to help people deal with work issues. But sometimes the person simply isn't ready, they're too affected.'

'Yes, people can sometimes need a break, space to be away from it before they can begin to reflect on what has happened and explore themselves and decide what to do next.'

'I think sometimes people can see counsellors too quickly. I suppose, in a way, as a person-centred counsellor maybe I can offer a space that doesn't have, I don't know, such a therapeutic agenda. What do I mean by that?'

'I don't know, but it seems important. Something about the approach that carries less of a therapeutic agenda? No, that doesn't sound right.'

'No, the agenda is there, but there may not be the pressure to have to resolve something coming from outside the client, in other words, from the counsellor.'

'Because of the non-directive nature of the approach, respecting a client for how they need to be, even if that is flat on their face with no motivation to get up, as it were?'

'Something like that, yes. I think that's what may be different about what we offer, and maybe others offer the same as well within other approaches, I don't want to sound as though as "we do it best", but I think that maybe there is a special something that is linked to the importance of accepting, unconditionally, how the client is, how the client needs to be. I really think that is different. Yes, I want to see people well, of course I do, but I don't know what is the best path for them to achieve wellness, do you know what I mean?'

'Mhmm, yes, you don't know what path they need to take, and I'd add, when they need to start taking it.'

'And maybe being allowed to be as they need to be, accepted as they are, and their experiences accepted and heard, you know, really heard. I'm sure that my eyes, my facial expression would have been reacting to the despair and at times sadness that was in Gerald's voice. And that can only be there when you are really attending. It's not there the same when you are sitting there trying to decide what is the best intervention to use, what is going to help this client feel differently, you lose it, you lose contact. I mean, you don't but in a way you do, and psychological contact or just simply contact is the first condition for constructive personality change according to person-centred theory.'

'So, having your thoughts on something else, even if you are listening and have eye contact, affects the quality of the contact. That makes sense.'

'So that's why I think the person-centred approach is different. Because the counsellor or psychotherapist, whatever term you use, isn't sitting their making plans, isn't having to think about what to say, they are fully attentive and then they respond with what they have heard, what has impressed them, or sometimes what they note has emerged from within themselves in response to what has been said. That's the difference, and I don't think it gets enough focus.'

Colin sat thoughtfully for a moment or two, he had been listening carefully to Barbara's words, and to the passion in her voice. 'And I'm just checking my own process here. Yes, I was listening to your words, and it was triggering off thoughts as you spoke, but if I had dwelt on those thoughts I would have lost you. I have to stay with you and then, when you have finished, see what is with me and respond out of that.'

This is an intriguing dialogue that is capturing something important about person-centred working. Giving the client full attention is vitally important, maintaining a sense of responsiveness to not only what is being said but also to the person themselves. As the client describes and communicates what is present for them, they do so in the context of a relational experience with the therapist. He is feeling heard as he speaks. This goes beyond feeling heard because of the counsellor's empathic response. That's a delayed sense of being heard. The one that perhaps really matters is the experience of being

> heard in the moment of speaking. That is a subjective sense, but will be encouraged by eye contact, facial expression, posture and a sense that tells us when we have someone's full attention.

'So we really do listen to our clients, really listen to them, and we trust that we will respond, I was going to say "adequately", but that doesn't sound good enough, trust that our words will reflect our sensitivity and responsiveness to what the client has said, and convey our empathic understanding or apprecia-tion of what has been disclosed, our unconditional positive regard and warm acceptance for the person and for how they are experiencing themselves and in a manner that is genuine, authentic, congruent and the client experiences that.' Barbara felt quite pleased with how she had put that. It was one of those moments when she wished she had had a tape recorder running.

'Can I quote you on that?' Colin had picked up on Barbara's smile of what he sensed to be satisfaction when she had finished her definition of person-centred practice. There was humour in his voice.

'Yes, you can, just make sure you spell my name right!' They both laughed.

'Seriously, though, I really do appreciate what you have just said. There is some-thing about the way the approach requires us to attend to our clients, and to not worry about our response until the space and time opens up for that responding to occur, and then we bring what is present for us, in that moment, into the dialogue we are having. It's something to ponder on further, I think.'

Barbara remained in touch with her passion for what she had said. She knew that there were no doubt times when she maybe didn't listen quite as attentively as she might, and she needed to watch out for experiences in herself arising that obstructed her listening which she brought to supervision – but the key to effective therapy was in listening and being sufficiently self-aware and empathically sensitive to communicate what the counsellor has experienced or is aware of in response to what the client has disclosed or communicated.

The supervision session moved on to a consideration of work with other clients.

Points for discussion

- Evaluate Barbara's effectiveness in terms of offering the core conditions.
- What enabled Gerald to begin to move into a more forward-thinking frame of mind?
- Were there times in the dialogue when you would have responded differently to what Gerald had said. If so, where, what would you have said, and why?
- What might you have taken to supervision had you been Barbara?
- How do you react to the exploration regarding contact and the particular sig-nificance of listening and attending within the person-centred approach?
- Reflect on your own practice. When a client is speaking, or is in silence, what percentage of your awareness is focused on listening to and attending to them?
- Write notes for the counselling session.

CHAPTER 10

Counselling session 2: making changes and the stress of working in the NHS

Three weeks later and a lot had happened. The counselling session seemed to have come at the right time for Gerald, and the holiday. He was back at work and had made some changes to his routines and had had some long discussions with his wife. That hadn't been easy. But things had now eased between them and he really didn't want that to change back to how it had been. But the work still flowed through, the need to keep on top of waiting times, produce reports and figures, deal with the fall-out from incidents. Somehow the job just didn't seem very satisfying any more. It was something he wanted to talk through with Barbara. He didn't feel comfortable talking to his manager about his disquiet over his job, didn't want him to think he was thinking of moving on. He wasn't sure himself, but for the moment he just needed to talk it through some more. He had discussed it with Maggie, and she was supportive of his thoughts of needing something different, and maybe a complete change; although he had worked for the NHS for many years and didn't want to compromise his pension.

He was also feeling anxious about Agenda for Change and the work it was causing him – having to redraw job descriptions and evaluate competencies. He had a lot of different staff to have to go through this process with, and he hadn't got the first idea where he was going to find the time. Barbara had appeared whilst he was lost in his thoughts. He got up and followed her to the counselling room. 'So, three weeks since the first appointment, how do you want to use our time today, Gerald?'

'Well, things have got a bit better.' He described the discussions he had had with his manager and with Maggie. 'So, the result is that I have restructured my day. My emails are going to be screened by one of the secretaries so I don't have to worry about that. I'll be passed those that need my attention and I'll have booked time to go through them and decide on what responses need to be made. And that's working. It really has made me realise how much time I spend reacting to and initiating unnecessary emails.'

'So, dealing with emails, handing them over to another member of staff, has made a difference.'

'I'm sure most of the things you send emails about could actually wait for a booked meeting. OK, yes, there are some things that come up, and maybe in the past it might have been a phone call, but now you send an email, or someone sends you one and there seems to be this sort of expectation of an immediate response – and that may not be coming from them, maybe from me. I don't know. I mean, when I send emails I suppose I do expect to get an answer if I'm asking about something specific and, yes, I guess I expect it, or want it, as soon as possible, preferably whilst I'm still thinking about it.'

'So a pressure to react, to respond, and an expectation that is how it will be?' Barbara didn't use the email a great deal herself, and when she did she would just collect messages, she wouldn't necessarily respond straight away.

'Pressure. And I think it's addictive, I really do. I mean, I'm as bad at home. I check my emails more than I really need to. Why check them more than once a day? You only get post once a day, so why do I need to keep checking my emails? It's crazy. So I'm trying to do something about that as well.'

'So you feel you check them more than you need to?'

'I'm sure I do, and I've thought about it but I don't know why I do it. Habit, I guess. And it's nice to receive messages from people. I'm into classical music in a big way, and I am a member of discussion groups about pieces of music, new recordings, that kind of thing, and I find myself wanting to check if someone's replied to something I've said. These kinds of network discussions, I mean, they're great in one way, but I don't know, I get the feeling that some people must be on-line 24/7. I suppose they are now that we have these different schemes for paying for access. Some people always seem to respond straight away, as if they are sitting, waiting for someone to say something. I'm not as bad as that.'

'So, email gives you pressure at work and feels addictive at home.' Barbara didn't mention the music she realised, but somehow it felt like it was the email that was the main focus.

'Yes, so I'm going to contain that as well, give myself time to get involved in that, again, get some structure. If I was going to some music appreciation society – in fact I occasionally do – but I mean if it was available 24/7, would I actually go 24/7? No. No, I need to get some control and some perspective here, treat it a bit like an evening class, give myself a couple of evenings, maybe, to settle down and see what people are saying and respond, not keep dipping in and out. It would probably make my life easier and I'm sure it would make it easier at home.'

'Mhmm, so, structure it and it will make your life, and home life in general, easier.'

'And we are trying to make the effort to get out more, to actually make time to go to the theatre and concerts. We'd drifted away from that. Maybe occasionally at weekends, but somehow that got lost as well. So, yes, we're booking things ahead, getting ourselves on theatre mailing lists, making a point of checking the "what's on" section in the local paper. It's what we both want to do, but somehow we got ourselves into a place where we weren't doing it.'

'So, it seems as though you've been putting in a lot of thought and planning with your wife on this. Planning ahead, giving yourself things to do.'

'More than that, it's also about having things to look forward to. I really think the weekends had simply become like a kind of pit stop before you went off again on Monday, back round and round the circuit. I guess you stopped at the end of each day, but it didn't really feel like it. So we're trying to make changes. And, as I say, there's something about having something to sort of look forward to, I don't know but that seems important as well.'

'Sure, something to look forward to, something beyond the pressure of the present.' Barbara added her own interpretation because it was an idea that she had found clients discussing, how you can get so caught up in the present that the future just becomes an endless continuation of the present, and if the present feels like shit, what hope for the future? But Gerald was giving himself hope, giving himself things to look forward to and, hopefully, experiences to remember, to feel good about as well.

Gerald was taking a deep breath, 'yes, very much so.'

Barbara nodded, aware that Gerald had lapsed into a silence. She guessed that he had said what he needed to say on that particular topic and so she respected the silence and waited for him to bring whatever else he felt he needed to air.

Why do silences occur at certain points in the therapeutic exchange? The counsellor has introduced something of her own interpretation in her brief response. It is likely that some silences are connected with something being introduced that the client had not been thinking about, or feeling, causing them to have to stop and decide what to do with it. That may sound strange, but it is like eating a hot casserole and someone hands you a scoop of ice-cream. There will then be a moment of hesitation as you try to decide what to do with what you have been given. Of course, it has no direct relationship to what you are eating, but once you have come through the initial hesitation you can then decide to maybe put it to one side for dessert.

In a way, this happens in counselling when a counsellor introduces something that requires the client to take a moment to absorb. Sometimes, though, the silence, the hesitancy, can indicate that what has been said is not empathic to the client's focus, at other times it might capture just what they were thinking and hadn't voiced, or may shed that patch of light that helps them to grasp their experience in a way that immediately makes sense to them. The person-centred counsellor will be hesitant in introducing too much unless there is a genuine sense that it is emerging from the therapeutic connection with the client, rather than their own history, or what others have told them.

'So I hope that everything taken together will make a difference, but I can't help wondering if I actually want to change my job, my role. I've been managing clinical services for some years now, and I just wonder whether I need to move into something less clinical, if only for a bit, maybe something that is more purely business orientated – not that the NHS isn't these days, but that's more the domain of the business managers in some ways, although not exclusively so. But maybe I need to think about something like that.'

'Get away from the clinical and move more into, what, contracting, financial management?'

'Something like that, either in a hospital trust, or into a PCT, primary care trust. They seem to have management posts though many of them do have a clinical remit. I don't know.'

'So when you say "I don't know", there's a sense of wanting some kind of change, of wanting to maybe move over into a different managerial role, but there is uncertainty as to what the motivation is? Maybe I'm wrong, it's just how I'm hearing the "I don't know".' Barbara was feeling a bit tentative as she spoke, and it was one of those responses that once she had got into it suddenly felt she had lost her way and wasn't sure where she was heading. She guessed she must have missed something, or some idea of her own had perhaps muddied in some way the clarity of what Gerald had been saying.

'I guess I don't know exactly why, maybe it's one of the hopes that the grass is greener on the other side!' He smiled and Barbara responded similarly. He continued, 'but I know it will be demanding, whatever role I take on, that's the nature of it, but I know I'm not thinking about managing clinical services in quite the same way. I mean, I line-manage team managers and, OK, they are managers, but they are clinicians as well, and so I am very close to the clinical work. Well, I have to be; I run a clinical department, I have to think not only managerially but clinically. And there's a tension. There's always a tension.'

'A tension between the managerial and the clinical?'

'Yes. Different priorities, different agendas. In many ways it is the core of the NHS problem, I think.'

'So this tension between the clinical and managerial goes to the very core of problems in the NHS as you experience them.'

'I think so. I mean, in the past, I guess the clinicians ruled in many ways, and then we had the internal market, fundholding, the purchaser/provider split. Hospitals had departments set up to monitor contracts, GPs had managers to manage their funds and their purchases. Budgets became more and more of an issue. Clinical services were dependent on what the purchasers wanted – in theory, at least. Sometimes it worked out that way, other times the hospitals carried on as they always did and just spent the GPs' budgets, putting through so much activity. And after the first wave of fundholding it got tighter and tighter, the budgets were pared down. Then we had changes from health authorities, to health commissions, then I think it went back to health authorities, or did it jump straight to primary care groups? Anyway, there were then primary care trusts, or PCTs, and now, well, now we have foundation hospitals on the horizon. The PCTs are overspending, economies of scale mean they're probably economically unworkable, so I guess they'll be amalgamated into new authorities that manage healthcare provision over larger areas and, my cynical self says sometime in the future some bright spark will come up with the idea of calling them health authorities. The wheel goes around.' He shook his head.

Barbara listened to what Gerald had to say. She didn't know a lot about the history of the NHS in this way, so she didn't know the rights and wrongs of what Gerald was saying, but it was clearly a view that he had developed and she respected that.

'So, the same but different.'

'The difference is the focus on money and management, on performance management, targets and budgets. As a manager I need to run services to budget, but clinicians want to run services to meet demand, and the two simply do not always match. My view is they will never match, not whilst we continue to invest so much money in advanced technology yet lose sight of the basics of healthcare. Do you know, I read recently that more people die in hospitals from infection than are killed on our roads each year?' Gerald was on a roll. He did have deep-seated misgivings about the NHS, though he didn't often speak of them. He wanted it to work. He knew the benefits, he knew how a free healthcare system was such a civilised development, but he also knew that it was under strain.

Barbara was continuing to listen. Clearly, Gerald felt passionate about the NHS and clearly he wanted, needed, to say these things. Perhaps by airing them in this way would help him. It felt to Barbara that he was certainly speaking from both head and heart. 'So, you are left with a lot of thoughts, feelings, concerns, and that statistic made a deep impression on you.'

'It did. It really did. Sometimes you don't come across things like that, but these sort of comparative figures can make you really question what is going on.'

'Mhmm, so you are left with lots of questions.'

'And another concern is how we survive as well on doctors and nurses from overseas. They make up such a large proportion of staff. And that's fine, I have no problem with people from overseas working in the NHS, but what of the countries that they have left behind, what do we do to the healthcare systems of other countries when we deliberately advertise and encourage so many to leave and come here?' He shook his head. 'It's the British way – take what we need without thinking about the consequences. It's the attitude of empire all over again.'

'You've got some strong feelings on the way it feels Britain takes from other countries.'

'And I'm not sure why I'm saying all this now, here, but yes, I have. I want services to be available. I don't want to be two nurses down on a Friday or Saturday night shift because of budgetary constraints. And, yes, I want the junior doctors to work more acceptable hours in the week; not the crazy situation we had in the past, but with less staff available how do we maintain services?' Gerald paused, and pursed his lips. 'Maybe I get too close, maybe I take it too personally, maybe I care too much, but that's how I see it. It frustrates the hell out of me.' He paused. 'And maybe that's another reason I get stressed.'

Barbara was aware of seeing a very different side of Gerald to the one she had seen three weeks previously, a man who then was feeling overwhelmed by his job, trapped, tired, needing space, a man who seemed to have hit a patch where he had barely enough energy to cope. A man in despair. Now, well, yes, another kind of despair, but anger and frustration and so much more energy. She noted her thoughts and responded to what Gerald had said.

'Frustrates the hell out of you the way it has become. This is a very different you I am seeing to how you were three weeks ago. And, as you say, maybe a contributor to stress.'

Barbara introduces her own experience of Gerald, highlighting the contrast. She uses her own experience, it is not something unrelated to the therapeutic dialogue although it might be argued that she is directing him towards her perception. It is a judgement that the counsellor has to make.

The person-centred counsellor will want to be responsive both to the client and to the reactions they experience being in the therapeutic relationship.

'I know. I know. But this is me.' He shook his head. 'I want to develop services, not constrain them, or cut them. I mean, I don't want to sound politically incorrect, but someone goes on long-term sickness – and I agree, staff have the right to that, of course they do, I have no problem with that, but is there funding to cover them in their absence? No. And so we have to do the best we can, or we go over-budget and the hospital has to cover it from somewhere else. At least we have some flexibility. There are other areas of the health service where I know for a fact that there is simply no money for cover, so that's it, services have to be cut or everyone else has to take on even more. I have a friend who manages substance misuse services. They are constantly juggling budgets, there is no slack any more, and they have had services come close to closure because of this very problem, particularly if you lose a doctor. Agency costs are almost double a normal salary, but there's no extra money to cover it.' Gerald took a deep breath and visibly sighed. 'Oh, I don't know. Not sure if talking like this does me any good. Probably just adds to my frustration.'

'That how it feels, leaving you even more frustrated.'

'Maybe not more frustrated, maybe more aware of the frustration that I already have.'

'I can appreciate that. So in a sense, talking like this puts you more closely in touch with what you really feel and think.' In other words, thought Barbara, it helps you experience yourself in a more authentic and congruent manner.

'Yes, for what good it does.'

'You don't think it does you any good?'

'Oh, I suppose it does, keeps me in touch with who I am and what I believe. I guess it adds to my determination to try and make the best of things. I know I talk about getting away from the clinical areas, but actually, well, maybe that's where I need to be. I guess I'd feel too remote spending all day monitoring activity in departments I had no influence over, negotiating contracts, checking budgets and expenditures.' Gerald shook his head, yes, he thought to himself, part of me would like to get away from the management/financial and clinical divide, but anywhere else wouldn't have the same buzz to it. 'The problem with all of this is that I know, and the consultants know, that at the end of the day, however much the clinical need, if the money isn't there they cannot spend it – at least they shouldn't. So whilst clinicians will rightly complain at reductions in service – we don't like to talk about cuts in the NHS, and certainly not rationing – when we make reductions because of budgetary constraints they know that however much they complain if there is no further funding, well, that's it. Unless there are ways of reconfiguring existing services to somehow free up monies, and that's easier said than done.'

'So, your sense is that actually you want to stay in touch with clinical services, however much the stress and tension between management and clinical priorities.'

Gerald nodded. 'Yeah, I guess so.' He was shaking his head. 'You know, you've got me really fired up today, I don't know how you did it.'

Barbara didn't know either, it wasn't that she felt she had said anything or encouraged anything. She felt simply that Gerald had a lot of pent up frustration and, well, today it was coming out. Maybe by listening she had encouraged it, but that was what she was there for, to listen and to facilitate clients to express or be how they needed to be. She liked the idea that he was being more of what he felt was himself. The energy he was showing had clearly got buried, bottled up, lost somewhere amongst the battering of stresses and demands that had come his way over recent months. Maybe the genie was out of the bottle and, like most genies, once they were out it was damned difficult to stuff them back in again. And anyway, maybe genies simply weren't designed to be bottled up . . .

'Maybe it was the right time, feelings, thoughts that are important to you were ready to break surface, as it were. There are things you needed to say, things that are important to you.'

'Maybe the changes I've been making have helped loosen things up a bit as well.' He smiled. 'I wonder how my manager would have taken all of this. I think he has some similar views but he's good at keeping them to himself.' He stopped and shook his head again, slowly, deliberately, 'why do we do it? Why do we put ourselves through it?'

'Why do we put ourselves through . . . ?'

'Why can't we somehow get back to, I don't know, something simpler? The NHS is so complex, involves so many different professions. We have hospitals gaining more and more independence, and that's great if they can innovate and maybe save money and direct it into new services. But what of those who can't, who simply cannot make those kinds of changes, and are under financial pressure? They need the money being saved by the innovators just to maintain services. How do we circulate it back to areas of need? Otherwise, we'll end up with yet another division between rich and poor, between those who scrape through and those who have excess. We'll just see the extremes of capitalism mirrored even more within the NHS. It's like the star ratings, they bring in extra money if you can get enough stars, and that's great, but if things slip and you have that money invested in services and staff, and the next year it's taken away, what then? Massed redundancies? And what if, because of budgetary constraints, some of that money had been needed for essential services, what then? There's no scope for longer term planning. We need to be able to plan longer term. We need consistency in our budgets over a longer time-frame, so we can plan the services, plan the investment, know what is possible, not go from year to year not knowing how much will be available.' He stopped and grinned. 'I'm off again, aren't I.'

'These are important matters to you, Gerald, you look around you; you think things through and draw your own conclusions. You see things that frustrate you. Yet you feel powerless to influence policy – at least, that's how it feels given the way you are speaking.'

> Throughout this session, Gerald has spoken at times at length. Barbara has not tried to keep summarising what he has said. Perhaps a counselling skills course might encourage that, but in person-centred therapy there is no place for constantly pulling clients back over their trains of thought and feeling. The dialogue is a flowing process, the client moves as they speak. The person-centred counsellor may on occasions show empathy for that journey, but often what is powerful is to simply empathise with where the client has reached on their journey – in other words, respond to what has been said at the end, or a sense of the way a client has been left feeling as a result of their dialogue journey.

'All I can do is try and ensure we have the best service possible for our patients with the budget that we have, and at the same time ensure that our staff have a working life that can contribute rather than undermine their well-being. And that's quite a challenge. I mean – and maybe I'm being simplistic, I don't know the statistics – but why in a society that today should know more about disease and what promotes health, why do we seem to have more of a demand on health services than ever before? I know the ageing population has a part in that, but not exclusively so. And anyway, we have National Service Frameworks which aim to reduce death and certain diseases. We can't reduce deaths, we can only delay them, or shift the cause to something else. I don't want to be morbid, but are we also considering quality of life? Everything seems to focus on quantity of life, but what about quality?'

'Quality not quantity.' Barbara paused, she had noticed the time. 'We need to end soon, Gerald.'

'I've said a lot, haven't I? Not what I thought I'd talk about, but it feels good having said it. Maybe I'm not getting all my facts right, I don't know, I only see what I see, pick up on what I hear or read, but . . . No, I'd better stop, I'll be off again.'

'Do you think it has been helpful, how this session has developed?' Barbara wanted to check this out, and she knew it was for her own benefit. In a sense, she did trust that Gerald had been as he needed to be, and she felt she had given him her attention, listened and hopefully communicated acceptance and warmth.

'Yes, I do. It's left me feeling more determined not to be flattened again by it all, to keep myself focused and in touch with what really matters to me. I'm sure it's not that easy – come and sound off for fifty minutes and then head back and it's OK. I'm making changes, but this is an opportunity to air what I really feel, and I hope you don't mind, I don't suppose other clients do this to you.'

'You'd be surprised. Let's say you are not alone with your frustrations, but people have their own take on it.'

'I'm sure they do.'

'But to answer your questions, no, I don't mind. It was good to hear your passion. Yes, good to hear it.'

'Thanks for that. I really do appreciate it.' He paused. 'So, when do I see you again?'

'When do you want to?'

'In a way it was good having this break, having some space between sessions. I know I had the week on holiday, but maybe we could make it in two or three weeks, see how things are?'

'OK, I can go with either, though three weeks would be slightly later in the day.'

'What time?'

'Three thirty.'

'That's fine. Let's go with that.'

Gerald left, feeling quite energised. He hadn't talked about what he had planned to say, but, well, maybe next time. He was amazed how different he was feeling, but at the same time he was wary. He still had to deal with work, he still had to stick to his changes. Things had built up before and he needed to make sure it didn't happen again.

Barbara was making herself a coffee. She felt she had earned it. She sort of felt that somehow there was hope with people like Gerald around, if they could keep themselves in touch with that passion. She wondered what he might have been like if he had been on the other side of the management/clinical divide, as he called it. She was genuinely pleased that he had begun making changes and that communication at home had clearly improved. Yes, maybe he had sought help at the right time, before things had become even more out of control. She had to hope that this was the case. She could only imagine how it might have been if the situation had continued for a few more months, if the manager hadn't told him to take a break and encouraged the referral to counselling, hadn't acknowledged that something was wrong rather than trying to keep him going. She thought back to the electric circuit. It was overloaded and waiting to go bang. She didn't understand electric circuits and wasn't sure quite how the metaphor would run given her experience of Gerald today. She had a vague memory from school of something about resistance. Maybe he'd freed himself up to be more in touch with his passion. Maybe that reduced resistance in some way, stopped him over-heating. She wasn't sure. But there was no doubt that energies were now flowing more freely in Gerald, the challenge now lay in maintaining them.

Points for discussion

- Was this a therapy session? What are your thoughts on this?
- What in particular stands out from this session, and why?
- Evaluate Barbara's responses as a person-centred counsellor.
- Had you been Barbara, would you have responded differently?
- Did Barbara avoid getting caught up in a discussion?
- What are your views in response to Gerald's comments?
- What are the pros and cons for spacing out counselling sessions, or should there be a rigid adherence to weekly or fortnightly contact?
- Write notes for this session.

CHAPTER 11

Counselling session 3: priorities and prioritising

'I'm doing OK. That last session really did get me going. Of course, I lost some of it over the next few days, still very busy but I'm sticking to the changes I've put into place. And my manager is still being very supportive. So, all in all, it feels as though things are working out well.' Gerald was sitting in the counselling room, feeling pleased. He was maintaining some kind of control over his workload. Fortunately, the incident that had happened involving the drunk patient had been resolved. That wasn't going any further although he had organised a refresher course on restraint for staff. He wasn't sure it was absolutely necessary but in the circumstances it seemed the right thing to do.

The current issue on his agenda, though, was the Agenda for Change process. And he had been involved in discussion not only with his manager, but across services, as to how the Trust was going to handle it.

'Good, so you feel on top of things at the moment.'

'Pretty much, except for the Agenda for Change, although even that is beginning to feel less daunting now that I'm getting a clearer picture as to what it is all about.'

'So you feel that you understand it more?'

'I think I did before, but it was the process and the time that would be involved. But it seems that the competencies are going to be established centrally in the Trust, so E grade, F grade nurses, etc., will each have their expected competencies for the grade. Job descriptions will need to reflect that but as they have all been brought into line generally in the Trust over the last couple of years, that should be fairly straightforward. There are meetings for staff to attend to help them understand it a little better.'

Barbara nodded. She was aware of that. She'd had clients making reference to their concerns and uncertainties but it seemed as though the process was now much more underway.

'And then we get staff to produce what they think their competency levels are, and that will then be considered to be clear as to what they may need to develop to reach the competencies for a particular grade, and some may be seeking a higher grade. I say grade, of course it will be a new system with less pay-scales. I mean, it does make sense but it also seems that some lower paid staff may come off less well than some higher paid staff, and that can't be right. So I'm sure there will be a reaction against that, but the principle is good, just that some of the detail may need looking at again.'

'So, you feel less stressed by it now?'

'I think so. I mean, it will take up time, but my manager has indicated that he intends to be involved and give support in the process. It's one of those things, it has to be done so we have to make time for it.'

'You sound more accepting, somehow.' Barbara was struck by the way Gerald had been speaking.

'Well, what can you do? I mean, get it over and done with. I've been through it and looked at what competencies I think my job requires and how my skills match it. I suppose it's like everything, so long as my view coincides with my manager's, then all is OK. It's where there is a difference and there may then need to be negotiations involving people trained up to facilitate the process, and maybe union reps too, then I guess it might get messy. But I think for the staff I have responsibility for it should be, at least I hope it will be, fairly straightforward. But it's a big undertaking and when you think the number of hours people are going to be putting into this up and down the country, it had better work because it's a lot of patient contact time being lost.'

Barbara nodded, 'yes, let's hope so.'

The counsellor has shared her view rather than empathising with what has just been said. Had she responded with, 'the loss of patient time is what concerns you' she would have maintained the focus and perhaps Gerald may have explored this further, possibly as a result connecting more strongly with his thoughts and feelings.

Gerald paused, wondering what to say next. Yes, he did hope so. It felt like an end to what he had been saying. Yes, he hoped so. His thinking went back to what was going on in the office, and whether anything else had particularly troubled him over the last few weeks. But things had settled down into a more manageable routine. He was feeling more relaxed in himself. Still frustrated at times, but more able to accept his situation.

'I did talk to my manager about whether I needed a change of role. He wasn't surprised, and wasn't going to stop me. He asked if there was anything I was interested in. I said I wasn't sure. I had been thinking back to our conversation in the last session and, yes, whilst it is frustrating in some ways, I don't want to lose responsibility for managing a clinical department. We discussed whether I might want to go on any training, perhaps further my management qualifications in some way. I said I'd think about it. I'm not sure, it wouldn't be until next year now so I don't have to make a decision. He said it could go into my next Personal Development Plan at my appraisal, and then if I still wanted to pursue it, at least it was in the paperwork, so to speak.'

'So, further study, but you're not sure.'

'Well, I don't know, it's something else I suppose although I get time off to attend of course. But I suppose I'm not sure. I guess part of it is I'm uncertain whether I do want to switch to a different job, and I don't want to commit myself to something I suppose in case I then want to move on. I don't know. I haven't got to make a decision yet, I think I need to see how the next few months go.'

'Yes, no need to rush into anything at the moment.'

'No point. But I've been keeping my eye on the internal vacancies, and, well, maybe if something appeals. But I don't really know. I'm not looking for anything specific, just looking, I guess.'

'Just looking in case something comes up that appeals in some way.'

'It'll need to be interesting, I think, need to have some clinical connection, maybe a bit more money but that isn't the main reason. Trouble is, where I live, if I was to look for something at another hospital, or another primary care trust, it would involve more travel and I'm not sure that I want that either.' Gerald had been giving it a lot of thought and felt that he could end up making things more difficult for himself, particularly as things had eased. There wasn't really any pressure to change.

'So, you're not sure about extra travel, extra money's not a big issue, so there's a sense that it might be better to stay where you are . . .'

'. . . or move to something within the Trust or, as I say, consider something at the PCT, although that might take me away from working with the clinicians.'

'So it sounds like you've been thinking it through and are fairly clear about it now.'

'I think so. And I'm just so glad that things didn't get any worse before they got better.'

'Yes, it seems as though you caught it – well, caught yourself, I guess, in time.'

> In this instance, the counsellor's summary has summed things up fairly accurately. Gerald feels heard and understood, there is nothing more that he needs to say at that moment on the topic. He moves his focus on to the area that is next most pressing for him, where he is also aware of change for the better.

'Things have eased more at home. The idea of organising a kind of social diary has helped. And we're thinking of taking up a foreign language class – problem is we can't decide which. We thought it would be good to do it together, but I want to learn Spanish and Maggie wants to improve her French. So we haven't resolved that yet. But it's a good sign. I think it would be fun to learn something together. I think we need it, it would be good for us. Work and stress had got between us, no doubt about that.' He took a deep breath as he thought of how it had become, more of a stand-off than a relationship. And the children seemed somehow more co-operative now as well.

'Even the children seem different, they don't seem to be quite as much the belligerent teenagers that they were. I don't know, the place seems calmer now.

I think that the way I had become was affecting everyone, but I hadn't seen it. Guess I was too caught up in myself and my own problems, couldn't see beyond them.' He shrugged his shoulders.

'That's how it can get, so overwhelmed that everything else fades into the distance.'

'And then it feels too big a gulf, or you feel it's all impossible and that makes you sad and lonely, and you feel hopeless and desperate, and then you drink, and I was heading that way. I really can see it now.' Gerald meant what he said. He could see how things were heading, though at the time, well, he'd probably have denied it. But he was on another path now. He still had the odd beer, and whisky some evenings, but it wasn't a habit, it wasn't the routine that it had become. He was pleased about that.

'So, you can see, looking back, where you were heading.'

'I mean, I like to think that I'd have come out of it, but I guess I do wonder. I don't know much about it. I don't think I'd ever be an alcoholic, I think I'm too sensible for that.'

Barbara smiled to herself inwardly, as she thought of all the sensible people she'd worked with at an alcohol counselling centre a few years back, people who thought it could never happen to them, but the wrong experiences at the wrong time, no support and the discovery that alcohol made them feel better, or the pub gave them a place to feel at home in, and the slippery slope can so easily begin.

'You feel you are too sensible to let it happen.'

'I like to think so. But, well, I did let myself get into a bit of state, didn't I, and I guess I'd never have believed that would happen either. Makes you think. Makes you realise that you really do have to look after yourself.'

'Mhmm, you know what happened, how you were feeling and behaving.'

'Hmm.'

Gerald pondered on what had just been said. 'Down to us, down to me, to make healthy choices where I can, do what I have to in order to keep well.' He paused again. 'Well, this has played its part.'

'I'm glad it has made a positive contribution.'

'Which reminds me, do you think I need to keep coming. I mean, it's nice to get away, but, well, what do you think?'

'Well, there's a limit of six, as you know. As to how many you feel you want or need, I am happy to leave that up to you.'

'It's good to take the time out, even to just, I don't know, talk about what's happening, anything really. I guess things may come up and I might be glad to have the time here.'

'Well, I am happy to see you for six sessions. I know that things have moved on, and I guess that for me, if counselling helps to ensure that changes that you make become, if you like, sustainable changes, then that's justification enough. But I don't need justification, but maybe you do?'

'Well, that's it really. Can I justify coming here, sitting and chatting about things? In one way I'm not sure that I can when I think of all the things I need

to do – I was going to say all the *important* things I have to do, but this is about
me and my well-being, isn't it?'
'Mhmm. It is.'

The counsellor does not empathise with the 'can I justify coming here?', but
that comment has passed on the client's journey towards reaching his conclusion that counselling is about himself and his well-being. Rather she
affirms his conclusion. In a sense, empathising with the strength and tone
of voice as he affirms what the counselling is for. Doubt is put aside in the
client's mind. And a component to this will be how he feels at having made
the decision. The counsellor has left it quite open for him to choose, and to
claim for himself what he feels he needs, wants, maybe deserves. It is a self-
affirming moment for the client.

'I think I'll keep coming, and the three-week gap works well. Weekly would be too
much. But to know I can come here another three times, that's, what, nine
more weeks, two months just over, that somehow feels good to know. Yes, I
guess it's like a safety net, you get to a point where perhaps you feel you don't
need it, but it's also kind of good to know it's there.'
'And I hope you don't need to use it for that purpose, but I'll leave it for you to
decide how you want to use this time.'
Gerald thanked Barbara. He then spoke a little bit about his children, how important they were to him, what they were doing in their lives, how he felt he hadn't
really spent enough time with them in recent years, something he regretted
and was determined to put right, although they seemed to be developing their
own social lives as they got older. He also went back to talking about how he
had become and what kind of role model he must have been, particularly for his
son. He said how he felt he wanted to have a chat to him about it sometime,
help him to realise how easy it is to make mistakes, let things get away from
you. He wanted to be sure that his son knew that he could turn to him if he
needed to, if he ever had problems. And he realised he wanted to communicate
the same to his daughter as well.
'We live in a stressful world and a stressful society. I don't know why, you'd think
with so much leisure and entertainment we'd all be a bit more relaxed about
things.' Gerald was being reflective. 'So much more going on these days than
when I was a lad. Funny, I remember being bored and my father telling me that
in his day they made their own entertainment. In a way so did we, but maybe
not as much. But today, I don't know, maybe I'm not being fair, but I think
there is a culture of "needing to be entertained", of a kind of dependency on
others meeting our needs, or it always being someone else's responsibility.
Sometimes I say things to my kids and I realise I'm saying what my father said
to me. That makes me smile. But there seems so much more pressure these
days, the commercial world, targeting young people all the time – have this,

buy that, anything and everything to make you look cool or feel happy. So much pressure. And if you can't afford it, what do you do, rob people or chase your highs in some other ways, joy-riding, drugs . . .' He shook his head. 'I need to spend more quality time with them. It's about priorities, and what really matters.'

Barbara nodded. As he was speaking she was reminded of an article she'd read some while back that had suggested that stress wasn't always something to manage, but could be seen as a necessary feature of human experience in a world that was out of sync. with the more human, some might say spiritual values, that often were a feature of people who wanted to spend their lives helping others. She made a mental note to look it out if she still had it when she got home.

The session drew to a close and they arranged the next appointment for three weeks time.

Barbara found the article when she got home.

Stress: A Heartfelt Necessity?

We hear the word stress mentioned increasingly these days. A great deal of ill-health is linked with high levels of stress. It may stem from home life: the children, relationship difficulties with a partner or family members, a move of house, an elderly relative to care for. Or it may originate in the NHS workplace, from NHS pressures: overwork, inadequate working conditions, unrealistic deadlines, lack of support/supervision. Stress may originate through change imposed on us from the outside, or through movement within our own natures. Change involves uncertainty that can cause stress. What will it be like? How will things turn out? How will I be affected? Will I be OK? We seem conditioned into experiencing a need to know what is going to lie ahead of us, even though we know that life is uncertain.

How might we define stress? Stress is defined in *Chambers Dictionary* as: 'a "constraining influence" and "system of forces applied to a body".' I would argue that stress is the effect of having to do something that you do not want to do, or of being required to do what you like doing, but for periods of time that are excessive. In a work situation you are given a task that you feel inadequate to cope with, or which you simply don't want to be party to, or have no time for – it doesn't seem that important – but are unable to say no. It may even be something you enjoy doing, but not for twelve hours a day. Stress is an effect of an imposition that is overloading your capacity to fulfil what is demanded of you and preventing you from doing what you really want to do. You are constrained by external forces that impinge on your personal time and space.

Stress is also an indicator of boundaries. We each have weak points that tell us we are under stress: backache, headache, irritability, insomnia, lack of motivation. We can build a picture of what we are comfortable with in our sphere of life, and what we find stressful. We can sense which external influences encourage a sense of fulfilment, and which diminish and disempower us. It puts us in a strong position to choose a path through life. It is certainly rare to feel completely stress free.

Heartfelt stress

We need to ask if there is a deeper cause, a deeper dissatisfaction with life and the experience it gives us. Is there a prevailing stress across societies that emerges from some deeper, human experience? Are we stressed by clinging to habits and ways of being and of functioning that block the inner nature of the heart from finding expression? Are we experiencing an increasing inner tension and flow of energy that has no outlet? We might call this 'heartfelt stress'. 'Heartfelt' (I have considered the use of the words 'spiritual' or 'humanitarian') is used to denote something at the core of our being, our essence, something deeply human, suggestive of a quality of stress arising out of inner processes that are concerned with individual spiritual growth and development and feelings of connectedness with others, and for many, with the planet.

Assuming, then, that stress is induced when the heart nature is obstructed from finding expression, how can we look at the suffering of humanity with open and sensitive hearts whilst finding ourselves pushed into behaviours that to some degree collude with separateness without feeling stress? We drive our cars and pollute the air. We invest our money and find it invested in turn in unethical activities. We buy the highly packaged food from the superstores and signal our agreement with their policies. We eat food that originates from the cash crops that the poorer countries have to grow to pay the interest on their debts to the world banking system, and to the very banks we invest in and whose profits we benefit from.

This heartfelt sensitivity as a cause of stress produces all kinds of effects on our natures. These may take physical form in disease; they may induce an imbalance in nervous energy and a feeling that nature can be thrown severely off-balance. It can produce a disorientation in our thought life, generating chaotic thought processes that distort our interpretation of what occurs in and around us. Heart energy is powerful.

Perhaps, though, we need to put aside the thought of getting rid of stress, or of seeing it as something to avoid. It is inevitable. We can use it to learn about our own capacities, recognising the signals we each receive when stress is building up. Then we can look for constructive recreation, to give our systems time out to re-energise, for instance through contact with nature. Meditation works for some. Simple communion with fellow human beings can also help.

If stress is the effect of a build up of energy (perhaps that energy is love) that is blocked from expression by our natures, then we need to seek ways of expression that are rewarding and creative, that lift our spirits. We might want to change our environment for a while, seeking resonance with the sounds of nature rather than the all too familiar noise of car engines, tyres on roads, and electronic clicks and buzzes. Perhaps part of our stress stems from not having enough of the range of natural vibration around us.

Dealing with stress can only be done on an individual basis. There is no universal panacea. Methods will differ from person to person, and the cause of the stress and the degree of sensitivity to the heart nature will be a crucial factor to consider. The heart-centred individual acknowledges the need for stress and learns to ride it, rather like a surfer rides a wave. He or she will use it to discover inner points of tension from which they can draw inspiration in their life and work.

The heart is calling us. We ignore her at our peril. If we do she is sure to ensure that the stress of circumstances will arise that will force us to draw her more fully into our lives.

Supervision session 2: passionate about the NHS

'So you are going to offer the full six sessions then?'

'Yes, I think it will help Gerald to consolidate, and it is still relatively early days and he may well need a bit of space to explore anything that may come up that is difficult or troubling.'

Colin agreed, 'and you let him decide?'

'I did. As a person-centred counsellor, what would you expect?'

'Well, you may have had a strong view.'

'I think it's important for people to take responsibility, yes?'

'Very much so.'

'And he needs to trust his own judgement and needs to know that others trust it as well. I would have accepted whatever he decided, though I hoped he would go for the six. I just think it's an opportunity, but he has his own meanings and his own priorities. But saying yes to the sessions is an acknowledgement of a need, or at least of a want, and as he said, it's important to him as a person, to his health and well-being.'

'Yes and I am sure that having made one decision for himself like that, it will help to strengthen him in making other choices as well.'

'I think so.'

Colin wondered how Barbara was feeling. She had already described the last two sessions and he was very conscious that much of it was about what Gerald had been saying, and not much about the effect on his supervisee. 'So, how about you, how has it been for you listening to what Gerald has had to say?'

'It's been interesting. It really has. In a way, it hasn't felt so much like counselling, at least not as some might see it, but he's using the therapeutic space the way he wants to, and I am staying with him on that.'

Colin was still aware that he had no sense of Barbara's feelings, but maybe it hadn't been so much a feeling contact with this client as a thoughtful or mental contact. He decided to share this as he thought it might usefully inform the supervision process.

'It seems that the last two sessions have involved more of a thoughtful focus than a feeling-orientated focus. Maybe it left you more aware of your own thoughts rather than feelings?'

'That's interesting.' Barbara sat and thought about it. 'I think you're right, although Gerald was certainly passionate about his ideas about the NHS. And that did feel good, felt alive. He could have got me motivated, I have no doubt, the way he was speaking. It was good to hear. I think I told him that.'

'Good to hear his passion for the NHS?'

'Yes, I mean, I do hear it from clients, and it is good to hear, but there was something about Gerald, particularly as a non-clinician. You sort of expect it from clinicians, but, well, managers are managers, but he seems to have a real passion for managing a clinical environment.'

'And that surprises you?'

'I don't know, maybe it does. I mean, I do see people who are literally doing what they do because they have to have a job. I guess I find that harder. I suppose because, as a counsellor, I'm on the clinical side, if that's the right way to put it.'

It seemed to Colin that an important issue was coming to light, the attitude of his supervisee towards clinical and non-clinical staff. He wondered, therefore, how it might be affecting the service that she offered. 'So you mean you have some kind of, I don't know, affinity with clinical staff? That may not be the right word.' Colin knew he sensed something but also that he wasn't quite sure what the right word was for it.

Barbara thought about it. 'I'm not sure. It seems to me that, well, maybe it's not that simple. I think it's probably more about attitude, and it's an attitude I see a lot of and maybe more on the clinical side, maybe ...' She hesitated, she thought of a number of administrative staff, secretaries, PAs, who had really conveyed an enthusiasm for their work and a real desire to get the best for their patients.

'So what I'm hearing is that there are those whose attitude has more passion about the NHS, about patient care, would that be right, and then in contrast others who simply see their work as a job, and they have to have a job?'

Barbara nodded. 'Yes, yes, and, well, if I'm honest I think I have to say that I do favour those who have that commitment to patient care, to making the NHS work.'

Colin nodded. It was a new issue for him to explore with a supervisee, but he could well appreciate the difficulty. 'So, I am still wondering, I guess, how this affects your practice.'

Barbara nodded as she thought about it. 'I hope it doesn't, but ... And it is a but, isn't it? I need to do some self-monitoring on this. I mean, I don't think I'm different, but if I am feeling different then it's very likely that I may come across differently, perhaps feel warmer, maybe be more encouraging to those whose attitude appeals more. Mhmm, I think we've unearthed something important here. And the NHS is, of course, an emotive workplace, not the same as some manufacturing business, say. Mhmm.' Barbara was concerned and intrigued. She was grateful that it had been picked up and she did need to think about it and keep an eye on herself. She began to reflect on recent clients, but it was difficult to get a sense of being different. She took a deep breath as she cocked her head to one side and looked up towards the ceiling. 'You know, I really think this is quite a significant issue, and not just for me, but generally. I wonder how other counsellors have dealt with it in the NHS.'

'It looks like something you really want to think about.'

'I do, and I'll bring it back and see where else I can go with it because it does feel important to me.' She shook her head, 'strange really, I mean, I've been involved in the service here now since it began and I've not thought about this, not specifically in terms of the NHS. I mean, we had problems. I wasn't seeing you, was I, when it began?'

'No.'

'No, but, well, it really took some work to get people to understand what we meant by confidentiality. Human resources, occupational health, and managers wanted to know what was happening for people they had referred. That was a mistake, accepting referrals from other professionals. We changed it to self-referral. It helped, but it took time, and even now, we still get phone calls: "I believe you are seeing . . . How's s/he getting on?''. We're used to it now and neither deny or confirm anything about anyone. But confidentiality and the health service, it is a nightmare, or at least it was as far as we were concerned.'

'Must have been quite a challenge to be involved in establishing the service.'

Barbara nodded. She was aware that time was passing and she had other clients she needed to discuss. She moved the focus on, but not before asking Colin to pay close attention to how she described clients from now on, in case there was anything in the style or content of her presentation that might link to that issue of whether she related differently to clients depending on their level of commitment to the NHS and patient care.

Points for discussion

- Was it 'right' for Gerald to be allowed to decide on whether he wanted all six sessions?
- What thoughts and feelings were you left with after reading session 3?
- Were there moments in the dialogue when you would have responded differently?
- How do you react to the notion of 'heartfelt stress'?
- Were there other issues that should have been brought to supervision?
- Given the notion that a client may receive a different response from a counsellor because of their attitude towards the NHS and patient care, how would you set out to deal with the problem?
- Write notes for the counselling session.

CHAPTER 12

Developments

Gerald attended session 4, reporting that he was maintaining the changes but that his workload was increasing again. He was trying to maintain his structures but they were under pressure. And he mentioned he wasn't sleeping too well again, work on his mind. But he hadn't resorted to drinking, he was maintaining his home routine. But he knew he was feeling more irritable and tired. Over the course of the week following that session he realised he was struggling and following a discussion his manager referred him to the Occupational Health Department.

He saw a nurse advisor there the following week, and found it helpful. He discussed what he was feeling, his heightened anxiety and general feeling of not being able to deal with what was coming his way. He had lost a team leader to sickness and hadn't anyone with enough experience to really act as cover, and he had no funding to bring someone else in. The nurse advisor wrote to his manager, suggesting that there needed to be a reduction in workload, and a temporary reduction in working hours and that whilst they understood the situation, changes had to be made as the situation was clearly affecting Gerald's health.

As a result, Gerald's boss had clearly made representation at a more senior level and arrangements were made to bring in another nurse as cover, and monies were found elsewhere in the system by the financial department. The hospital could not afford for the Accident and Emergency Department to be carrying the heightened risk. They were aware that it was being run very much on the edge, it had been highlighted in a process that had taken place earlier in the year when all sites had produced 'Risk Registers', highlighting risks and potential risks under certain headings or categories, such as health and safety, resourcing, clinical. The shortages in resourcing had been noted as being a high-risk factor given the lack of flexibility for funding to cover any long-term paid absence.

The fifth session was spent reviewing the current situation. Gerald had been allowed to pass on some of the Agenda of Change responsibility. He had felt some relief, it had been proving more time consuming than he had anticipated. Gerald once again spoke about wondering whether he needed a break from the department, something new, something different. Barbara noted a sense that his passion was ebbing once more, and she commented on this. Gerald had agreed, realising that he needed to try and contain his work so that it didn't get back into his family life once more. He'd made the telling remark, 'bottom line is, family comes first. I lost sight of that before, but not this time.' He left the session very much with this in his mind.

Counselling session 6: moving on

'I took a few days off, got away for a few days, I needed it, the family needed it. And I've decided to look for another job. I will stay in the NHS, and I am prepared to travel if necessary. I just have to look after myself. It's not that they are not trying at work, they are, but I know that within me I've lost it. I don't look forward to going in any more. I regained it but have lost it again. Maybe I'll get it back, but I can't go on yo-yoing like this. And actually, making that decision has made a difference. It's like, I seem more able to cope now that I know it won't be forever. I mean, I always knew it wouldn't be forever, but now I feel like I've changed the timescale. I guess I've been toying with this ever since I started coming here, but when things got easier I pushed it away. But it's been around, I guess. So, I'm looking. I won't rush into something for the sake of it, that's not the answer, I know that, but I think I need something where I can experience a bit of freshness. I think you get stale. Same issues come around again and again. Same weekly and monthly routines. No, I need something fresh. Something, somewhere where I think I'll be able to feel more fulfilled, where I can get back in touch with that sense of doing a good job, rather than running from one thing to the next.'

Barbara sat listening to Gerald as he spoke. He seemed very sure in what he was saying. It felt like he had given it a lot of thought. 'Feeling you're doing a good job is important to you, not just feeling you're running from one thing to the next.' She made her empathic response to the final thing that Gerald had said, wanting to communicate that she had heard him, but minimising the risk of disturbing his flow.

'It's not that I think the job is impossible, I don't think that, but maybe all that has happened has made me think differently, made me more aware of my own needs. And, yes, maybe I do have different priorities now. Work isn't everything. Yes, it's important, but I'm fortunate, and if necessary I could earn a little less and we could get by. But I'm not planning on that at the moment.' Gerald did feel clearer in himself once he had realised what he wanted to do, and it had become a want. He wasn't reacting against circumstances, he felt it as being more of an orderly retreat. Nothing wrong with that. No, he wanted to stay in control, make his own choices. He'd do his job, and do it to the best of his ability, but he wasn't thinking long term and he was going to put family first. He'd spoken to his manager who said he understood and hoped he would change his mind, but that he would support him in whatever he felt he needed to do. He quite agreed that Gerald needed to look after himself, that he had, in many ways, held the service together and kept staff motivated in a very effective way.

The focus moved on to consider the next steps. What were Gerald's needs now that the counselling was coming to an end? What support did he feel he needed?

'I've thought about that, but I feel quite clear in what I need to do. The things that Maggie and I are doing – getting out more, having more of a life as a family – that is making a big difference. But if I have problems, can I refer myself back?'

'That's no problem. Obviously, hopefully, you won't need to, but the service is here. And I'd be happy to see you again.' Barbara was glad that as part of the deal on accepting a six-session maximum number of sessions it was agreed that there was flexibility around how soon someone could be seen again if they needed to re-refer. Barbara generally encouraged people to have a break long enough to experience how it was without the counselling. Where there was a specific issue that was on-going and non-work related, something that had emerged through the counselling process, then she would encourage her client to seek counselling elsewhere. Part of her contract was that she couldn't see someone herself. She understood the reasons for this, but felt it was unfortunate. Clients built up therapeutic rapport with their counsellors, and vice versa, and she believed that there should be the possibility for people to continue to see the same counsellor privately. But she knew it was not unusual and she certainly knew that many employee assistance programmes which offered counselling services to organisations had that condition in their agreements with counsellors. She had her view, she knew others felt the same, but that not everyone agreed. She felt there was a lack of understanding of the nature of the therapeutic relationship as *a*, if not *the*, key factor in effective therapy.

The session drew to a close with Gerald expressing his appreciation. Barbara said that she really valued and appreciated his passion for the NHS, and also felt saddened that it was being squashed by the demands made upon him, but that she also felt so good that he felt he was able to make choices and decisions that put his own well-being and his family relationships first. 'So it's a mix of feelings that I'm left with.'

'Well, for me it has certainly been timely. I feel like I had fallen down and hadn't been able to get up, then I got picked up and you were part of that, then I stumbled again, fell but this time I've picked myself up, and now, well, it's like maybe the path is too bumpy, or slippery, or something, and as I can't flatten it out or make it more stable, I have to find another path.'

Barbara nodded. What a wonderful piece of imagery. She voiced her thoughts. 'That is quite an image. So now, find a flatter path.'

Gerald nodded. 'One that I can keep my feet on.'

Barbara was struck by Gerald's sense that he had picked himself up this time. That seemed crucial. 'And you know, now, that you can pick yourself up.'

'Yes, but I'd prefer to avoid falling over!'

Barbara smiled, 'yes, quite.'

'So, thank you, thank you for listening to me, to my ramblings, my ups and downs. Thank you for being flexible in letting me come every few weeks, I've taken a lot from it.'

'I'm pleased. So have I. I've learned more about the stresses in middle-management and of your passion for the NHS.'

'That won't go away, and neither will I! I'll find something.'

'I'm sure you will, and I'm not just saying that, I believe it. Anyway, the time has arrived, so you take care of yourself, I feel that you will.'

'You too, thanks again.' The session ended. Gerald left feeling positive about his future even though he knew that the decisions he had made meant short-term uncertainty, but life was uncertain. He liked the idea of being open to possibilities. He was moving on, he didn't know when, or to where, but it felt timely.

Points for discussion

- What were the significant points in the four sessions described here?
- What impression do you have of Gerald? Using your words, describe him as a person and, if you know someone else who has read the book, ask them to do the same. Then compare what you have written. Discuss why differences in your descriptions might arise.
- Critically evaluate Barbara as a counsellor and supervisee. What are her strengths? What do you feel are her weaknesses?

Reflections

Barbara's reflections – 'I'm sorry that Gerald is moving on, but I feel that wherever he goes, he will do a good job, he will bring his heart into his work and want to ensure patients receive an excellent service. I've enjoyed working with him. I still feel I didn't say a great deal. Gerald is quite a talker. But he seems to have talked his way along the therapeutic journey to find a place from which he can make choices that he feels to be right. To me, that's a successful outcome.

'This raises an interesting issue, of course. How do we judge a successful outcome of workplace counselling in the NHS? Staff staying in their jobs and knuckling down to it in spite of the demands? Staff deciding they need to do something else? Staff re-prioritising and putting their well-being or job satisfaction higher on their list of priorities?

'It leaves me wondering what it is that we are offering as staff counsellors in the NHS, whatever our employer or the nature of the organisation whose staff we see. Are we offering therapy which, as we know, can take a person to unexpected places where they find themselves making decisions that were not anticipated when they started the counselling process? Or are we offering emotional support to help someone simply keep going? Or a bit of both? Or something else?

'As a person-centred counsellor I offer therapeutic relationship defined by the presence of the "necessary and sufficient conditions for constructive personality change". Constructive personality change – some people speak of therapeutic change. But do I set out to change people? Well, people come because they are struggling with something and that generally means there is some degree of incongruence – experiences being denied to awareness. Maybe we could say that Gerald was denying to his awareness the fact that he was experiencing his job as overloading him, or perhaps that he was denying to his awareness the need to make different choices in his life, the need to make changes.

'I cannot go into a session with an agenda. But I don't know that managers in the NHS will always see it like that. Investment in a counselling service is to invest in a system to ensure that they get a maximum return on the NHS staff members. The NHS wants them "made better" and back in the workplace doing a good job, maybe a better job. Or is that a bit cynical? For me, where a client is doing the work that they want to do, and feeling valued in that work and fulfilled in what they are doing, then they are going to be a more effective employee. And if counselling means that they realise that this job does not satisfy them, does not bring them a sense of feeling valued, then maybe it is in everyone's best interests for them to choose another path. Of course, it is hoped that the staff member will feed this back to managers in the hope that adjustments can be made, though it may not always be possible.

'I produce six-monthly reports detailing the issues being brought to counselling. No names, but I also give a breakdown by gender and by ethnicity. The Trust wants to know what is stressing employees and this communication is part of its strategy for improving the working lives of its staff. Of course, Improving Working Lives is an initiative that contributes to star ratings and extra resourcing, so it's important for many reasons.

'I wish Gerald well. I am sure he has made the right decision. It hasn't been a knee-jerk reaction. He's thought it through thoroughly.'

Gerald's reflections – 'I'm sharing my thoughts and feelings and it is now two weeks after the last counselling appointment. I'm still determined to move on and I have applied for another job that came up, actually in the local mental health Trust. I haven't worked in mental health, so I may not get an interview, but it struck me that it would broaden my experience and somehow it just appealed. As I was writing the application form, there was the usual section for a supporting statement. I got thinking and remembered a friend from many years back who had suffered with depression and sadly killed himself. Somehow, it came back to my mind and I remember feeling, yes, I really did want to understand mental health services. We have a duty psychiatrist at the Accident and Emergency Department and a psychiatric liaison service. I've obviously been aware of that component of Accident and Emergency but somehow, filling in the application form and remembering what happened to poor Roger, I don't know, I felt a kind of burst of enthusiasm, and I felt quite emotional as well. I still feel it as I sit here sharing my thoughts. I think I really do want that job.

'So, we shall see. I think I talked rather a lot in the counselling. I don't know if that was what I was meant to do, but that's me. I guess I've always had a lot to say. I always think that being a communicator is one of my strengths. But that session when I talked about my feelings for the NHS, yes, that was important. It really did help me to get back "me". I'm a passionate man, I guess. I don't want to just have a job or do a job. It has to have some purpose, some meaning, I want to go home and feel my day's been worthwhile; not just shuffling papers around and looking busy to justify a salary. Not that there's time for that anyway, but my work is important to me. I do believe there is something vocational about working for the NHS, and I think that somewhere that's been lost. But I don't want staff exploited for that sense of vocation either, I've seen that too. Back to that clinical/managerial relationship.

'At least Clinical Governance brings us all around the table. Those meetings really have made a difference, giving us a forum to discuss matters across specialities and professions. I know our meetings in Accident and Emergency involve representatives from each relevant profession, plus managers and administration as well. It really brings people into the decision-making process, although there are still areas where there are differences that are difficult to resolve and, yes, generally it is a case of "the budget rules, OK!". But not always, clinical cases are made for extra funding, to ensure service provision is not diminished and where possible we do try to find extra resources to develop new services. Not easy in a culture of CIPs – cost improvement performances – having to do the same with less. OK, to begin with, but as time goes on you hit that critical point at which services are threatened. We haven't been there, not quite anyway, but I know it happens elsewhere in the NHS.

'One thing I hope to see is for our department, and all A&E departments to be funded for specialist alcohol counsellors or nurses, to deal with the rising levels of alcohol-related admissions. That new Alcohol Harm Reduction Strategy (for England) seems to highlight the need, but doesn't seem to have any money for a service that seems to me to be so basic and fundamental.

'I'm digressing. I said I talked too much. The counselling. Yes. Well, if things get on top of me again, I'd certainly go back for another chat. I still can't really put my finger on how it helped, but it did. Having time out? Someone without an agenda? That surprised me, I expected the counsellor would be pushing me in some way to get myself together, but it wasn't like that at all. I had time. I was listened to. Well, I probably didn't give her a chance to say much! But Barbara did listen. She looked like she wanted to hear, that was important, yes, the way she looked, the way she sat there. She probably didn't need to say much, I knew she was listening, and I somehow knew she wanted to listen. Makes me smile, I guess she has a vocation for what she does, not something you just do as a job. Hmm, yes, that was important. Funny, isn't it, just someone sitting there and giving you time, but it's more than that, I'm sure. She's trained, and yet, I don't know, can you learn to listen like that? Or is it something you either have within you, or you haven't?

'I'm speculating on something I know little about, but it does make me think of my work and my staff. How little time they get to listen to people. OK, maybe that's more appropriate in other areas of healthcare, but it's so important. I guess they have more time in mental health services, they must have, it must be so important for the patients.'

Author's epilogue

At the end of most of the *Living Therapy* books that I have written I am left wondering how the clients' lives will turn out. Of course, they are purely fictional, but they always seem so alive somehow. And they say such interesting things. They get me thinking, and I'm just the one that writes down what they think and feel!

This book has been close to my heart as someone who has experience of both clinical and managerial responsibility within the NHS. Not that I have specifically drawn from my personal experience, but I am aware of issues that arise, of difficulties and challenges, of stresses and tensions, and in the course of my work I have met people working in many different areas of healthcare.

The NHS is a multi-cultural employer, perhaps more than any other, which is so refreshing. It enriches the organisation, but that doesn't mean there aren't racist issues to be addressed and examples of oppression. But the NHS is also an organisation under stress, and this affects people at an individual level. At the end of the day I believe strongly that an organisation's stress manifests in the health of its staff members. And stress can tease out deep-seated prejudices that people may not even be aware of. The NHS is a learning environment, and most importantly a place where we learn about ourselves.

The NHS has been subject to constant change certainly since I first joined a GP surgery in Guildford to enter data on to the computer system in preparation for its entry into the fundholding system (in the early 1990s). And I know that changes were already in process, but for me, from that time on, it seemed that nothing stayed still. Whilst the aim of all the change is to improve services, (and cost-saving), it nevertheless affects staff who, however committed they are, can reach breaking point. And often it seems those who are most committed reach that point. Maybe, some of those without the same commitment to the NHS have already left and found something else to do that is more fulfilling or less demanding, perhaps realising that they have to put their own health and family life first.

I certainly believe that NHS staff who have shown commitment to the NHS are all champions, and anyone who survives over ten, twenty, thirty years should certainly be recompensed and their achievement acknowledged, although I know many such people would simply wish to be left alone to get on with their jobs. That says a lot in itself. It was timely that as I was writing this book the film about Patch Adams (starring Robin Williams) came on the TV, reminding me of his work. I met Patch many years ago at a Medical Marriage Conference in

Findhorn, bringing allopathic and complementary practitioners together to dialogue and explore. I believe in his message of wellness and believe it has to be established within the culture of the NHS. He writes of the healing power of love and laughter (Adams, 1993). He brings medicine and clowning together. Patients need healing, so do staff. And we all need to feel that our NHS is a work setting in which we can feel well and encourage wellness.

I welcome the Improving Working Lives initiative in the NHS, but it needs to go so much further. Think of an organisation as a person, each hospital trust as an organism. What will make that trust evidence healthiness? What would be the evidence for the presence of wellness? Well, feeling empowered to look after itself, to make choices that are satisfying, ensuring that it exists for a purpose, that it has the freedom to act in accord with serving that purpose, and that the purpose is achieved to an acceptable degree.

There is no place for racism and oppression in a healthcare system, no place for empire building, for individuals and services exerting power over others. When a cell in a body does that we call it cancer. Specialities must be allowed to specialise, to serve their particular function within the body of the health service, but not in isolation. There needs to be feedback and learning, cross-discipline exchange. The NHS is a system, and a 'living' system because what makes it alive are the people involved, the staff members *and* the patients. The patients give it a purpose, the staff members respond to that purpose. Whilst in a brain-like way priorities and standards must be directed centrally, movement and development must also take into account sensory information entering the system – through staff contact with patients, through the experience of procedures followed and outcomes measured.

In his Foreword to Patch Adams' book, *Gesundheit!*, Matthew Budd writes that 'inauthenticity is our modern form of plague: it kills life' (Adams, 1993, p. ix). Person-centred counselling encourages authentic living. It helps people get in touch with who they are, helps them find their own passion. Counselling services for staff members in the NHS should serve this purpose, enabling people to become or reclaim who they authentically are so that they can make a difference to the lives of others, whether they are the clinician directly treating patients and with time to connect on a human and heartfelt level with the people they care for; or the receptionist who has the time to remember to smile because they are genuinely pleased that the patient has attended.

I hope you will have enjoyed reading this book. Whilst it has addressed therapeutic issues it has also engaged with organisational and political matters. But that cannot be avoided. The NHS workplace is a political arena, and people will bring opinions and beliefs into the counselling sessions. I am sure you will not agree with everything that I have written; all I ask is that you consider the importance of ensuring the mental, emotional and physical health of staff members – their wellness. Achieving this is, in a very real sense, a successful outcome in the running of a healthcare system. Staff members – clinical, administrative and managerial – that feel well are probably more likely to have a positive effect on the patients, and on each other.

It is my view, no, let's be authentic here, it's my passionate belief, that person-centred counselling, and the philosophy of human relationship that underpins it, has a part to play in contributing to authenticity and wellness in the NHS workforce.

Appendix 1

The Gesundheit! Institute[1]

Our mission

To bring fun, friendship, and the joy of service back into healthcare.

Our vision

The Gesundheit! Institute is dedicated to upholding a radical socio-political vision replacing greed and competition with generosity, compassion and inter-dependence.

1 As a stimulant to broaden the healthcare delivery dialogue, Gesundheit! Institute's mission is to build a hospital/healing community and provide care based on these principles:
   - all the healing arts are welcome
   - all patients are treated as friends
   - there is no charge for health services
   - no third-party reimbursement is accepted
   - the healthcare experience is infused with fun
   - no malpractice insurance is carried by the Institute
   - the health of the staff is valued equally with the health of the patients
   - the health of an individual is nested in the health of family, community, society and the natural environment.
2 We seek to stimulate caring by encouraging grassroots, neighborly mutual support and personal activism.
3 We aim to animate community health responsibility by assessing community health needs and resources, mobilising and inspiring a right relation between

---

[1] Gesundheit! Institute, P.O. Box 3134, Hagerstown, MD 21741–3134, USA. http://www.patchadams.org

153

these, and nurturing a snowball effect of activism that supports sustainability of individual and community health.

4   Pioneer, through research, the understanding of the implications of the healthy interdependence of personal activism, mutual support, vibrant community and world peace.

References

Adams P (1993) *Gesundheit!* Healing Arts Press, Rochester, US.

Borrill CS, Wall TS, West MA *et al.* (1998) *Stress Among Staff in Trust's Final Report.* Institute of Work Psychology, University of Sheffield, Sheffield.

Bozarth J (1998) *Person-Centred Therapy: a revolutionary paradigm.* PCCS Books, Ross-on-Wye.

Bozarth J and Wilkins P (eds) (2001) *Rogers' Therapeutic Conditions: evolution, theory and practice.* Volume 3: *Congruence.* PCCS Books, Ross-on-Wye.

Bryant-Jefferies R (2003a) *Counselling a Recovering Drug User: a person-centred dialogue.* Radcliffe Medical Press, Oxford.

Bryant-Jefferies R (2003b) *Time Limited Therapy in Primary Care: a person-centred dialogue.* Radcliffe Medical Press, Oxford.

Bryant-Jefferies R (2004) *Counselling for Progressive Disability: person-centred dialogues.* Radcliffe Medical Press, Oxford.

Bryant-Jefferies R (2005) *Counselling Victims of Warfare: person-centred dialogues.* Radcliffe Publishing, Oxford.

Coles A (2003) *Counselling in the Workplace.* Open University Press, Maidenhead.

Department of Health (2000) *The Provision of Counselling Services for Staff in the NHS.* Department of Health, London.

Embleton Tudor L, Keemar K, Tudor K *et al.* (2004) *The Person-Centred Approach: a contemporary introduction.* Palgrave MacMillan, Basingstoke.

Evans R (1975) *Carl Rogers: the man and his ideas.* Dutton and Co., New York.

Gaylin N (2001) *Family, Self and Psychotherapy: a person-centred perspective.* PCCS Books, Ross-on-Wye.

Haugh S and Merry T (eds) (2001) *Rogers' Therapeutic Conditions: evolution, theory and practice.* Volume 2: *Empathy.* PCCS Books, Ross-on-Wye.

Kirschenbaum H (2005) Carl Rogers' life and work: an assessment on the 100th anniversary of his birth. *Journal of Counseling and Development.*

London Hazard Centre (1999) 'Bullying at Work'. LHC Factsheet. http://www.lhc.org.uk

Mearns D (1999) Person-centred therapy with configurations of self. *Counselling.* **10**: 125–30.

Mearns D (2000) The nature of 'configurations' within self. In: D Mearns and B Thorne (eds) *Person-Centred Therapy Today.* Sage, London.

Mearns D and Thorne B (1988) *Person-Centred Counselling in Action*. Sage, London.

Mearns D and Thorne B (1999) *Person-Centred Counselling in Action* (2e). Sage, London.

Mearns D and Thorne B (2000) *Person-Centred Therapy Today*. Sage, London.

Merry T (2001) Congruence and the supervision of client-centred therapists. In: G Wyatt (ed.) *Rogers' Therapeutic Conditions: evolution, theory and practice*. Volume 1: *Congruence*. PCCS Books, Ross-on-Wye, pp. 174–83.

Merry T (2002) *Learning and Being in Person-Centred Counselling* (2e). PCCS Books, Ross-on-Wye.

Patterson (2000) *Understanding Psychotherapy: fifty years of client-centred theory and practice*. PCCS Books, Ross-on-Wye.

Rogers CR (1942) *Counselling and Psychotherapy: newer concepts in practice*. Houghton Mifflin, Boston.

Rogers CR (1951) *Client-Centred Therapy*. Constable, London.

Rogers CR (1957) The necessary and sufficient conditions of therapeutic personality change. *Journal of Consulting Psychology*. **21**: 95–103.

Rogers CR (1959) A theory of therapy, personality and interpersonal relationships as developed in the client-centred framework. In: S Koch (ed.) *Psychology: a study of a science*. Volume 3: *Formulations of the Person and the Social Context*. McGraw-Hill, New York, pp. 185–246.

Rogers CR (1967a) *On Becoming a Person*. Constable, London. Original work (1961).

Rogers CR (1967b) The interpersonal relationship in the facilitation of learning. In: R Leeper (ed.) *Humanizing Education*. NEA, Washington, DC, pp. 1–18. Reprinted in: H Kirschenbaum and VL Henderson (eds) (1990) *The Carl Rogers Reader*. Constable, London, pp. 323–34.

Rogers CR (1980) *A Way of Being*. Houghton-Mifflin Company, Boston, MA.

Rogers CR (1986) A client-centered/person-centered approach to therapy. In: I Kutash and A Wolfe (eds) *Psychotherapists' Casebook*. Jossey Bass, San Francisco, pp. 236–57.

Royal College of Nursing (2002) 'Working well' survey. In: *Counselling for Staff in Health Service Settings: a guide for employers and managers*. RCN, London.

Tudor K and Worrall M (2004) *Freedom to Practise: person-centred approaches to supervision*. PCCS Books, Ross-on-Wye.

Warner M (2002) Psychological contact, meaningful process and human nature. In: G Wyatt and P Sanders (eds) *Rogers' Therapeutic Conditions: evolution, theory and practice*. Volume 4: *Contact and Perception*. PCCS Books, Ross-on-Wye, pp. 76–95.

Wilkins P (2003) *Person-Centred Therapy in Focus*. Sage, London.

Williams S, Michie S and Pattani S (1998) *Improving the Health of the NHS Workforce. The Report of the Partnership on the Health of the NHS Workforce*. The Nuffield Trust, London.

Wyatt G (ed.) (2001) *Rogers' Therapeutic Conditions: evolution, theory and practice*. Volume 1: *Congruence*. PCCS Books, Ross-on-Wye.

Wyatt G and Sanders P (eds) (2002) *Rogers' Therapeutic Conditions: evolution, theory and practice*. Volume 4: *Contact and Perception*. PCCS Books, Ross-on-Wye.

Further reading

Association for Counselling at Work (1996) *Counselling Skills and Counselling at Work: an introduction for purchasers and providers*. ACW, Rugby.

Berridge J, Cooper C and Highley-Marchington C (1997) *Employee Assistance Programmes and Workplace Counselling*. Wiley and Sons Ltd, Chichester.

Carroll M (1996) *Workplace Counselling: a systematic approach to employee care*. Sage, London.

Carroll M and Walton S (eds) (1997) *Handbook of Counselling in Organisations*. Sage, London.

Cooper CL, Allinson T and Reynolds P (1989) Stress counselling in the workplace: the post office experience. *The Psychologist*. **2**: 384–8.

Cooper CL and Sadri G (1991) The impact of stress counselling at work. *Journal of Behaviour and Personality*. **6(7)**: 411–23.

Cunningham G (1994) *Effective Employee Assistance Programmes*. Sage, London.

Department of Health (2001) *Improving Working Lives: national audit instrument*. HMSO, London.

Employee Assistance Professionals Association UK (1998) *UK Guidelines for Audit and Evaluation for Employee Assistance Programmes*. EAPA, Rugby.

Employee Assistance Professionals Association UK (2000) *UK Standards of Practice and Professional Guidelines for Employee Assistance Programmes*. EAPA, Rugby.

Hardy S, Carson J and Thomas B (eds) (1998) *Occupational Stress: personal and professional approaches*. Stanley Thornes, London.

Health and Safety Executive (2000) *Securing Health Together: a long-term occupational health strategy for England, Scotland and Wales*. HSE, London.

Health and Safety Executive (2001) *Tackling Work-Related Stress: a managers' guide to improving and maintaining employee health and well-being*. HSE, London.

Health and Safety at Work (1974) *Health and Safety at Work Act 1974*. HMSO, London.

National Assembly for Wales (2000) *A Human Resources Strategy for NHS Wales: delivering for patients*. National Assembly for Wales, Cardiff.

National Assembly for Wales (2001) *Improving Health in Wales: a plan for the NHS with its partners*. National Assembly for Wales, Cardiff.

National Health Service Executive (1998) *Working Together: securing a quality workforce for the NHS*. HMSO, London.

National Health Service Executive (2000) *The Provision of Counselling Services for Staff in the NHS*. HMSO, London. Also available at the Department of Health website: www.doh.gov.uk/nhscounsel

Royal College of Nursing (2002a) *Working Well Survey*. RCN, London. Also available at the RCN website: www.rcn.org.uk

Royal College of Nursing (2002b) *RCN Guidance on Traumatic Stress Management in the Health Sector*. Also available on the RCN website: www.rcn/org.uk

Royal College of Nursing (2002c) *Working Well: a call to employers*. RCN, London. (To order a copy quote publication code: 001 595.)

Scottish Executive Health Department (1999) *Towards a Safer, Healthier Workplace: occupational health and safety services for the staff of the NHS in Scotland*. DoH, Scotland.

Scottish Office Department of Health (1998) *Towards a New Way of Working: the plan for managing people in the NHS in Scotland*. DoH, Scotland.

Useful contacts

Person-centred

Association for the Development of the Person-Centered Approach (ADPCA)
Email: adpca-web@signs.portents.com
Website: www.adpca.org

An international association, with members in 27 countries, for those interested in the development of client-centred therapy and the person-centred approach.

British Association for the Person-Centred Approach (BAPCA)
Bm-BAPCA
London WC1N 3XX
Tel: 01989 770948
Email: info@bapca.org.uk
Website: www.bapca.org.u

National association promoting the person-centred approach. Publishes the journal *Person-Centred Practice* and a regular newsletter *Person-to-Person*.

Person-Centred Therapy Scotland
Tel: 0870 7650871
Email: info@pctscotland.co.uk
Website: www.pctscotland.co.uk

An association of person-centred therapists in Scotland which offers training and networking opportunities to members, with the aim of fostering high standards of professional practice.

World Association for Person-Centered and Experiential Psychotherapy and Counselling
Email: secretariat@pce-world.org
Website: www.pce-world.org

The Association aims to provide a worldwide forum for those professionals in science and practice who are committed to, and embody in their work, the theoretical principles of the person-centred approach first postulated by Carl Rogers. The Association publishes *Person-Centered & Experiential Psychotherapies*, an international journal which 'creates a dialogue among different parts of the person-centred/experiential therapy tradition, supporting, informing and challenging academics and practitioners with the aim of the development of these approaches in a broad professional, scientific and political context'.

Workplace counselling

Association for Counselling at Work (ACW) – a division of BACP
1 Regent Place
Rugby CV21 2PJ
Tel: 0870 443 5252
Email: acw@bacp.co.uk
Website: www.counselling.co.uk

BMA Counselling Service
Tel: 0645 200 169

Provides a telephone counselling service.

British Association for Counselling & Psychotherapy (BACP)
1 Regent Place
Rugby CV21 2PJ
Tel: 0870 443 5252
Email: bacp@bacp.co.uk
Website: www.counselling.co.uk

Confederation of Scottish Counselling Agencies (COSCA)
18 Viewfield Street
Stirling FK8 1UA
Tel: 01786 475140
Email: cosca@compuserve.com
Website: www.cosca.org.uk

Doctors' Support Network and Doctors' Support Line
Tel: 0870 765 0001
Websites: www.dsn.org.uk and www.doctorssupportline.org

A self-help organisation for doctors with, or who have recovered from, mental illness. Includes a telephone helpline.

National Counselling Service for Sick Doctors
Tel: 0870 241 0535 (helpline).
Website: www.ncssd.org.uk

Provides independent, confidential advice from doctors to sick doctors and their colleagues when ill health may be impairing safe medical practice. The NCSSD works within the usual ethical framework that governs all doctors.

RCN Counselling Service
Royal College of Nursing
20 Cavendish Square
London W1G 0RN
Tel: 020 7647 3464
Website: counselling@rcn.org.uk

RCN Direct
Tel: 0845 772 6100

24-hour information and advice for RCN members.

RCN Nurseline
Royal College of Nursing
20 Cavendish Square
London W1G ORN
Tel: 020 7647 3463
Email: nurseline@rcn.org.uk
Website: www.rcn.org.uk

UK Council for Psychotherapy
167–169 Great Portland Street
London W1W 5PF
Tel: 020 7436 3002
Email: ukcp@psychotherapy.org.uk
Website: www.psychotherapy.org.uk

Index